101 Tips

FOR THE PARENTS OF

GIRLS WITH AUTISM

101 Tips

FOR THE PARENTS OF

GIRLS WITH AUTISM

The Most Crucial Things You Need to Know about
Diagnosis, Doctors, Schools, Taxes, Vaccinations,
Babysitters, Treatment, Food, Self-Care, and More

Tony Lyons

Contributions by Kim Stagliano

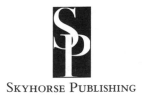

SKYHORSE PUBLISHING

57059347

616.85882
LYO

Skyhorse Publishing books may be purchased in bulk at special discounts
for sales promotion, corporate gifts, fund-raising, or educational purposes.
Special editions can also be created to specifications. For details, contact
the Special Sales Department, Skyhorse Publishing, 307 West 36th Street,
11th Floor, New York, NY 10018 or info@skyhorsepublishing.com.

Skyhorse® and Skyhorse Publishing® are registered trademarks of
Skyhorse Publishing, Inc.®, a Delaware corporation.

Visit our website at www.skyhorsepublishing.com.

10 9 8 7 6 5 4 3 2 1

Library of Congress Cataloging-in-Publication Data is available on file.

Print ISBN: 978-1-62914-508-2
Ebook ISBN: 978-1-62914-842-7

Cover design by Eve Siegel

Printed in the United States of America

WARNING: The information contained herein is for informational purposes only. Neither the editor, nor the publisher, nor any
other person or entity can take any medical or legal responsibility of
having the information contained within *101 Tips for the Parents of
Girls with Autism* considered as a prescription for any person. Every
child is different and parents need to consult with their own doctors, therapists, lawyers, financial advisors, or other professional to
determine what is best for them and their child. Failure to do so can
have disastrous consequences.

Contents

Introduction

What are little boys made of?
Snips and snails, and puppy dogs tails
That's what little boys are made of!

What are little girls made of?
Sugar and spice and all things nice
That's what little girls are made of!

What are autism parents made of?
Courage and care as we pull out our hair
That's what autism parents are made of!

I was sitting at my small and always cluttered computer desk in the eating area of my kitchen (ah, the glamour of being a writer) when I received a call from Skyhorse Publishing. They asked if I would take a book of 1,001 tips for parents of girls with autism, compiled by publisher Tony Lyons himself, and cull the tips for a new book.

As Mom to three daughters with autism, I do have certain bona fides when it comes to females on the spectrum. My girls are not youngsters any longer, so I have a pretty long view of their autism. I have the experience of having weathered school and puberty and the terror of starting to face post-school adult issues. My daughters, whom you met in my 2010 memoir *All I Can Handle: I'm No Mother Teresa*, are now twenty, eighteen, and fourteen.

I am inordinately fond of the Skyhorse Publishing team for their commitment to the autism community and sheer bravery in presenting autism related topics and authors to readers. Publisher Tony Lyons has a beautiful daughter on the spectrum (you can read about her in *Finding Lina: A Mother's Journey from Autism to Hope*, her mother's book) and he has melded his love for Lina with his passion for publishing.

For those of you who are familiar with my writing and who may follow me on Facebook or Twitter, you know that one of my best stress relievers is standing in my kitchen and whipping up something savory or sweet. Cooking and baking are outlets for me as an Italian American "Mama!" and autism Mom. You also know that I'm all about "the retro"—seems I was born at least a decade later than I should have been. I collect vintage cookbooks, and while I'm not above using a King Arthur Flour gluten-free boxed mix on a regular basis, I also love scratch cooking and baking.

So when asked to do this book, I without hesitation said, "Yes! I'd love to create a recipe for success for parents of girls with autism!" I danced around the kitchen for moment, excited at the prospect of a new book. "This will be a piece of cake!" Aha! I had found my theme and format for this revised version of a book that, in its original format, is like a huge multi-tiered cake. One thousand and one tips is a lot of info! This book is more like a table set with platters of *petit fours*. Small bites to get you started as you look for info to help your own daughter, loved one, student, patient, or client with autism. I've sprinkled recipes into each chapter, just for fun. Some I've adapted from my favorite cookbooks (with references, of course) and others are from a terrific book from Skyhorse called *The Autism Cookbook: 101 Guten-free and Allergen-free Recipes* by Susan K. Delaine, a fellow autism Mom.

In thinking about a book that's geared to females with autism, a Joe Jackson song popped into my head:

"Don't you know that it's different for girls . . ."

Autism is different for girls in many ways. Girls are expected to be social, to have better communication skills than boys, and to understand social cues, facial expressions, and feelings better than boys. Girls are expected to brush their hair, polish their nails, play with dolls, wear skirts and dresses, sit quietly, and play nicely.

Uh-uh. Not in my household, and probably not in yours. Outside of their beauty, my girls aren't very "girly" at all. Boys can get away with not having a full complement of social and communication skills—even without autism. You and I know that it *is* different for girls. That said, many of the strategies needed to navigate school, home, and the world apply equally to boys and girls.

As parents of daughters I think we need to be hyper-focused on safety. Let's face it: our kids tend to be ethereally attractive. What better victim than a gorgeous woman who does not have the ability to advocate for herself fully or, in many instances, to communicate any form of abuse? It's a harsh reality and a recipe for disaster. We've already lived it with my youngest, who was abused on the school bus in 2010. Criminal charges, a civil suit—agony.

I want you to think of the hard work you've had so far and the work you face in terms of creating the safest possible life for your girl. School? Raising a girl who can read even at a basic level and entertain herself quietly with books—from "I Can Read" basic books to chapter books to novels or non-fiction—is a challenege. Making sure that she can sit safely in the library or at a coffee shop looking completely typical—even more so. Toileting? An imperative skill. How many times a day do you use the toilet? Five times? Six times? A female who can tend to her own bathroom hygiene does not need another person to assist her. That's five or more times a day that her body is private and protected. Kind of scary to contemplate, but it's the reality.

The harder you work at getting skills into your girl at as young an age as possible, the bigger the payoff for her. But I'm here to tell you that our girls can gain skills forever. I have zero tolerance for the concept of windows and doors slamming shut. My daughters are not buildings. Neither is yours. I have seen them gain skills year after year. Sure, much of it is at a snail's pace, and some of the skills are at a five-year-old level. But you know what? Five-year-old skills are ahead of three-year-old skills. It's progress. Don't panic if your daughter doesn't have the skills you think she should have at her age—just keep plugging away. She will surprise and delight you.

Please bear in mind that each cook brings his or her own "touch" to the food. Three cooks with one recipe will turn out three slightly different dishes. The same holds true in autism. A tip that works for "Jane" might be a flop for "Susan." We'd all love a recipe for success for our girls. Use this book as a guideline to help you feel less alone in your journey to raise your daughter with autism.

Thank you to Tony Lyons and the incredible team of experts who wrote the original tips. The book begins with education. If you picked up the book based on the title, then you're past diagnosis day and likely looking to dig into a meal. I hope you feel that I have provided some sugar and spice, and that you'll read the book twice.

;)

KIM

CHAPTER 1

Education

If your daughter is under the age of three, you should contact your local Early Intervention program for access to services including speech, OT, PT, and more. These are free services, and many times the therapist will be able to come to your house. When we started Early Intervention in Bucks County, Pennsylvania, in 1997, Gianna was a newborn and getting out of the house was really tough. Google "Early Intervention" and the name of your state and/or county, or ask your pediatrician's office for a contact.

In 1986, Congress established a program of early intervention for infants and toddlers with disabilities in recognition of "an urgent and substantial need" to:

- Enhance the development of handicapped infants and toddlers and to minimize their potential for developmental delay;
- Reduce the educational costs to our society, including our Nation's schools, by minimizing the need for special education and related services after handicapped infants and toddlers reach school age;
- Minimize the likelihood of institutionalization of handicapped individuals and maximize the potential for their independent living in society;

- Enhance the capacity of families to meet the special needs of their infants and toddlers with handicaps.[1] (http://www.parentcenterhub.org/repository/ei-history/)

After the age of three, your daughter is eligible for early intervention services through your local public school district. These services can include a half or even full day of preschool, as I discovered in Hudson, Ohio, when we moved from Pennsylvania in 1999. Both Mia and Gianna qualified for the program by virtue of their Early Intervention evaluations. This is another reason to make sure you are "in" Early Intervention: to smooth the transition into school-age services. As an exhausted Mom of two young children with autism, the mere thought of a school bus picking up my girls and taking them for morning early intervention services was heaven on earth. Take advantage of any and all services you can as soon as possible for your daughter and for yourself. Self-preservation is as important as your daughter's progress. Trust me.

Resources:

Wrightslaw Special Education Law and Advocacy
www.wrightslaw.com

Parents, educators, advocates, and attorneys come to Wrightslaw for accurate and reliable information about

---

[1] Findings of Congress as stated in Public Law 99-457 (1986). P.L. 99-457 is the statute of the Education of the Handicapped Act Amendments of 1986, passed by Congress on October 8, 1986. Available online at: http://www.eric.ed.gov/PDFS/ED314927.pdf

special education law, education law, and advocacy for children with disabilities.

Begin your search in the Advocacy Libraries and Law Libraries. You will find thousands of articles, cases, and resources about dozens of topics. See more at www. yourspecialeducationrights.com. The site's primary purpose is to empower parents with the knowledge and understanding they need to advocate for their child's education through engaging video programs.

Know Your Rights!

yourspecialeducationrights.com is the first and only video-based resource for parents. The site was developed by Special Education Attorney Jennifer Laviano, Special Education Advocate Julie Swanson, and Mazzarella Media, one of the nation's leading educational content providers.

Never before have parents had the ability to learn about their rights in such a practical, user-friendly format. Members will have access to a continuously updated video library covering essential information in order to secure appropriate special education services for their child.

Jen and Julie's experience brings to members the perfect combination of perspectives as lawyer, advocate and parent.

IDEA: Your Child's Rights

Under the Individuals with Disabilities Education Act (IDEA), services such as speech therapy, occupational therapy, vision therapy, and behavioral therapy can be provided to the child by the school district, on the condition that it has been decided that it needs to be a part of the student's individualized program at an Individual Education Program (IEP) team meeting, and written into the IEP. Parents need to inform themselves about the school district they are in, the quality of the services, their rights, and which professional in the area is the best to provide assessments of their daughter.

—Chantal Sicile-Kira, www.chantalsicile-kira.com

~

IDEA was passed in 1990 and is designed to provide kids with learning disabilities an *appropriate* education in the least restrictive environment possible. Parents are to be partners in choosing the best education fit. To do this, parents need to become familiar with the law so they know their rights and what services are available for their children.

~

Parent rights under IDEA include the right to ask for an evaluation of your child at any time and the right to be part of the team deciding what special education services and therapies will be provided to your child.

~

IDEA provides for your child to have an Individualized Education Plan (IEP) designed for her specific needs; for example, how much occupational, physical, and speech therapy will be provided.

~

Should you not come to an agreement with your daughter's school system, you do have the right to a due process hearing where an administrative officer or judge rules. Should it come to this, you will require the services of a lawyer. Again, it's best to have an attorney (specializing in education law) in advance of this eventuality, if at all possible.

~

What's the big IDEA? It's important to know that IDEA is in effect for your child until she graduates from high school, or until she reaches the age of twenty-one; after this point, services are provided on a state-by-state basis. Under IDEA, every child is entitled to a Free and Appropriate Public Education (FAPE), regardless of disability. In this context, the US Supreme Court has taken *appropriate* to mean that the program "must be reasonably calculated to provide educational benefit to the individual child." In addition, under IDEA, all children are to be placed in the *least* restrictive environment possible. Remember: special education is a service, and *not* a place.

~

Here are the key parental rights under IDEA to remember:

- Parents have the right to be informed and knowledgeable about all actions taken on behalf of their child.

- Parents have the right to participate in all meetings regarding evaluation and placement.
- Parental consent is required for evaluation and placement.
- Parents have the right to challenge educational decisions through due process procedures.

~

The related services your daughter may be entitled to include:

- Speech therapy
- Occupational therapy
- Counseling
- Nursing services—medication administration
- Transportation
- Paraprofessional—health and/or transportation para

Tips for Achieving the Least-Restrictive Environment for Your Child by Timothy A. Adams, Esq. and Lynne Arnold, MA

Don't allow your child to lose out on the benefits of being educated alongside typically developing peers. The least restrictive environment (LRE) is a fundamental requirement of IDEA: *To the maximum extent appropriate, children with disabilities, including children in public or private institutions or other care facilities, are educated with children who are not disabled; and special classes, separate schooling, or other removal*

---

of children with disabilities from the regular educational environment occurs only when the nature or severity of the disability of a child is such that education in regular classes with the use of supplementary aids and services cannot be achieved satisfactorily. 20 USC § 1412(a)(5)

~

Remember that general education is the default placement. Before offering a more restrictive environment, the school district must consider what supplementary supports and services, accommodations or modifications would allow the child to be successful in a general education setting.

~

Don't be afraid to ask "why?" It's the school district's job to explain to you why its placement offer is the LRE for your child. The IEP team must review the continuum of placement options before determining which one is the LRE for your child. As the parent, you're the most important member of that team. Be sure to personally observe any proposed placement and consider bringing an independent evaluator with you.

~

Ask the IEP team to explain each time segment of your child's school day that has been designated as "inclusion" or "mainstreaming." Make sure that any time your child's IEP says she will spend among typical peers is meaningful. Otherwise, for example, your child's inclusion time during lunch may only mean that your child is in the cafeteria at the same time as the regular education children. Your child may be restricted to a special table or there may be no attempt to facilitate her interaction with general education students.

~

Consider the benefits of your child's exposure to same-aged peers who are modeling age-appropriate language, skills, and abilities. Children learn from each other and imitate each other. Inclusion can make a big difference for a child both academically and socially, and eventually determine if the child will be on track for a certificate or diploma upon high school graduation.

~

Don't accept excuses that general education with an aide is more restrictive than a special education classroom. By definition, LRE is determined by the child's exposure to her typically developing peers. If an aide is keeping a child from her peers, that's a training and supervision issue, not an appropriate rationale to keep a child segregated in a special education classroom.

~

Ask the IEP team about the implications of various placements. If the district says your child's needs will be best met in a special education classroom, make sure you understand the specifics of those supposed advantages. For example, although a special day class will typically have a higher ratio of teachers/aides to children, it's not a matter of simple math. Some aides may already be assigned to provide 1:1 help to specific children, and overall, the class may include children whose exceptional needs would skew the actual ratio throughout the school day. Also, the number of the children in the classroom can widely fluctuate throughout the school year.

~

Don't let unaddressed problems become an excuse for removing your child from a general education classroom. For example, if a child is disruptive, let's determine a plan for reducing and eliminating the problem behaviors, which often includes developing a behavior plan. It's an absolute inequity for an IEP team to simply move a disruption into a special education classroom. If your child's behavior is disruptive, why is it unacceptable for the general education classmates, but reasonable for the special education classmates to experience?

~

Don't allow your child's right to an individualized education program to be solely determined by the district's existing structure for special education placement. For example, districts often tell parents that a particular classroom or program requires a certain testing score or other subjective criteria. Just because your child doesn't fit neatly into their existing programs doesn't lessen their obligation under state and federal laws to meet her educational needs.

Remember the phrase "appropriate education." Your daughter is entitled by the Individuals with Disabilities Education Act (IDEA) to a free and appropriate public education. If your BOE cannot provide one, they must cover the cost of an appropriate private school. Appropriate does not mean best! Keep this in mind. *The Supreme Court interprets an appropriate education plan as one that "must be reasonably calculated to provide educational benefit to the individual child."*

~

Remember, services are expensive, and, because of financial pressures, your state would prefer to offer as little as possible—so be prepared to fight.

~

Should you believe a private school is the best option, and you'll miss the $60k to $100k they cost, you will need an education lawyer. EDUCATION LAWYER. Not Uncle Steve or your next-door neighbor who happens to be an attorney. For this you need a specialist. Ask your target school, as they likely have a list of lawyers other parents use. Interview a few and choose the one you like, and ask for parent references!

~

Be aware that parents have a lot of power. Don't wait for two months to check in for results. If something is not resolved quickly, work on it. Teachers don't always have as much leverage as you think. You may be able to help your child's teacher resolve something much faster. Work as a team.

—Autism and PDD Support Network,
www.autism-pdd.net/autism-tips.html

~

You and the district will have to come up with an Individual Education Plan (IEP). To prepare, read *The Complete IEP Guide: How to Advocate for Your Special Ed Child* by attorney Lawrence Siegel, and talk to parents already in the school system you are targeting to learn about what they have experienced.

~

Don't make assumptions. Small schools can offer excellent services, and large schools can offer poor services. Schools in rural areas can be enlightened. Schools in suburban districts can be stuck in outdated methods. Get to know your child's IEP team members, and keep an open mind. Sometimes teachers need to be educated about autism and are open to learning more if it means helping your child.

—Patti Ghezzi, schoolfamily.com,
www.schoolfamily.com/school-family-articles/article/
10685-help-your-autistic-child-succeed-in-school

~

Nothing is as important as making a personal visit on a normal working day, to a short-list of several schools. Do not take your child with you on these preliminary informal trips; she may become excited, confused, or agitated, especially if she visits several in a short span of time.

—Oaasis Information Sheet: Finding a Special
Needs School/Home Learning,
www.oaasis.co.uk/documents/info_sheets/
finding_a_special_needs_school

~

It is often an educational goal for parents and professionals for a child to be mainstreamed. While an important goal, it is more important to consider your child's feelings of competence in these settings. Typical role models can be good, but the reality is that children's interactions are full of innuendo. Academically, your child may be able to keep up with a mainstream class, but socially, she is likely lagging behind. Ask yourself: are these role models providing positive experiences for my child, or is my child feeling bullied, isolated, or incompetent in that environment?

—Laura Hynes, LMSW, RDI Program Certified Consultant, www.extraordinaryminds.org

~

Some questions to ask when you visit a recommended program:

- What is the educational philosophy of the program (ABA, DIR, TEAACH)?
- What is the class size and ratio to teachers/teaching assistants?
- How long has the school been using the current program (ABA, DIR, etc.)?
- How do the nonverbal kids communicate?
- What kind of success has the program had (i.e., kids moving to less-restrictive classes)?
- What programs are offered to parents?
- How long has the teacher taught at this school?
- What is their experience with kids with autism?
- How are related services provided?
- What services are currently being provided to students in the class?
- Does the school have a consultant or supervisor certified in the particular philosophy?
- Does the consultant/supervisor conduct ongoing training for school staff?
- What is the age makeup of the class? (There can only be a three-year age span in each class.)

- Where do the special education kids have lunch and recreation?
- Are there inclusion opportunities?
- How does the staff handle behavioral issues and/or self-injurious behaviors?
- What types of reinforcers are used at the school?
- Is medical staff available at the school?

Don't forget to observe a class and take copious notes!

~

It is illegal for a school to tell parents that their child cannot come back to school unless on medication!

Communicating with the School

Communication: The most important thing to do is to establish open communication. Try to be nonthreatening. You can make friends and get what you need.

—Autism and PDD Support Network,
www.autism-pdd.net/autism-tips.html

~

But if making friends doesn't work, prepare to fight!

~

Be sure to communicate any concerns or ideas right away, with a note, while the discussion can be relatively casual. By communicating early, you can avoid becoming angry and frustrated; by intervening early, you can avoid a situation growing into a bigger problem or crisis.

—Autism and PDD Support Network,
www.autism-pdd.net/autism-tips.html

~

Consider your options. When you're having a contentious experience with your child's teacher, or when you think your child needs more than the school will be able to provide, look into private therapy, which might be covered by insurance. If you aren't able to access services your child is entitled to, consider hiring an advocate or special education attorney to help you work with the school. Be the squeaky wheel that gets the grease.

—Patti Ghezzi, schoolfamily.com,
www.schoolfamily.com/school-family-articles/article/
10685-help-your-autistic-child-succeed-in-school

~

Whether a child with autism is in elementary, middle, or high school, the first step to fostering support begins with parents meeting with teachers and school leaders. Every public school is legally required to offer all students special services, and therefore, the earlier parents can meet with the school, the more tailored the program can be made for your autistic child.

—Grace Chen, "5 Tips for Helping
Your Autistic Child Excel in Public Schools,"
www.publicschoolreview.com/articles/88

~

As autism rates are soaring across the country, many schools are creating programs, classes, and resources specifically for students with autism. If the school does not offer these resources, ask leaders if any nearby cooperating county/district schools provide autism-specific support.

—Grace Chen, "5 Tips for Helping Your Autistic
Child Excel in Public Schools,"
www.publicschoolreview.com/articles/88

~

Document your child's condition and school requirements. If your child is diagnosed with an autism spectrum disorder, make sure that the school has a copy of the diagnosis. This might seem obvious, but in some cases the school and district have been able to point out that they were unaware of any actual diagnosis of autism disorder.

www.wellsphere.com/autism-autism-spectrum-article/
ta-tips-tips-for-securing-a-teachers-assistant-for-
your-autistic-student/146550

~

One very effective way to keep communication open is to use logbooks. The teachers (and others who are working with your child) write in these each day and send them back home with the child. The parent reads what the teacher(s) write and responds and sends the book back with the child. These are especially effective with nonverbal children. It keeps the communication open between parent and teacher(s). Plus, sometimes writing to a teacher makes it easier to communicate an idea exactly the way you want to express it.

—Autism and PDD Support Network,
www.autism-pdd.net/autism-tips.html

~

Inform teachers immediately of any unusual circumstances occurring at home. A stressed child cannot attend to tasks, often exhibits disruptive behavior, or might simply space out. Teachers might misread these signs. Examples range from divorce to a sick grandmother to a new baby. Each student has a very different response to these life changes.

—Autism and PDD Support Network,
www.autism-pdd.net/autism-tips.html

~

Make a list of things you want to say before you go to a meeting and take it with you. When you meet, give yourself plenty of time to discuss important issues.

—Autism and PDD Support Network,
www.autism-pdd.net/autism-tips.html

~

Ensure that the school has a "home base" for your daughter on the spectrum if she is mainstreamed or fully included—a quiet and safe place where she can go to review information needed for her class, or to cope with any stresses and behavioral challenges.

~

If there is a new teacher, this will of course be a considerable adjustment. Obviously, it would be helpful to meet this teacher (with just the child and family present) before school starts. To get a sense of expectations, it would be useful to know this teacher's rules as explicitly as possible before school starts.

—Lars Perner, PhD, www.aspergerssyndrome.org

~

If something is bothering me, I can . . . This visual card can be taped to the child's desk or placed in a small photo album with the following illustrated examples:

- Raise my hand for help
- Close my eyes and count to ten
- Take five big breaths
- Ask for a break

—Roger Pierangelo and George A. Giuliani,
Teaching Students with Autism Spectrum Disorders

~

When I was a child, loud sounds like the school bell hurt my ears like a dentist drill hitting a nerve. Children with autism need to be protected from sounds that hurt their ears. The sounds that will cause the most problems are school bells, PA systems, buzzers on the scoreboard in the gym, and the sound of chairs scraping on the floor.

—Temple Grandin, PhD, author of
Thinking in Pictures and *The Way I See It*,
www.autism.com/ind_teaching_tips.asp

~

The fear of a dreaded sound can cause bad behavior. If a child covers her ears, it is an indicator that a certain sound hurts her ears. Sometimes, sound sensitivity to a particular sound, such as the fire alarm, can be desensitized by recording the sound on a tape recorder. This will allow the child to initiate the sound and gradually increase its volume. The child must have control of playback of the sound.

—Temple Grandin, PhD, author of
Thinking in Pictures and *The Way I See It*,
www.autism.com/ind_teaching_tips.asp

~

Some children might need to be warned in advance about fire drills.

~

Some autistic people are bothered by visual distractions and fluorescent lights. They can see the flicker of the sixty-cycle electricity. To avoid this problem, place the child's desk near the window or try to avoid using fluorescent lights. If the lights cannot be avoided, use the newest bulbs you can get. New bulbs flicker less. The flickering of fluorescent lights can also be reduced by putting a lamp with an old-fashioned incandescent light bulb next to the child's desk.

—Temple Grandin, PhD, author of
Thinking in Pictures and *The Way I See It*,
www.autism.com/ind_teaching_tips.asp

RECIPE

Pizza Dough

Recipe adapted from Dom DeLuise's *Eat This . . . It Will Make You Feel Better*

- 1 package dry yeast
- 1 cup warm water
- 3 cups all purpose flour
- 1 tablespoon olive oil
- 1 tablespoon Kosher salt

Turn on the light in your oven. Dissolve the yeast in the warm water and stir until it foams. If you have a stand mixer with a dough hook, place the flour in the bowl, add the salt, olive oil, and warm water, and mix for 10 minutes until a smooth ball forms. No mixer? Place the flour on a double-wide sheet of waxed paper, make a well in the center, add the salt and olive oil, and then slowly drizzle in the water with one hand while mixing the water into the flour with the other. Gather the wet dough and hand-knead it for up to 15 minutes (it's therapeutic!), by which point you will have a smooth ball of dough. Place the dough into a large oiled bowl, cover with a slightly damp tea towel, and place it in your oven with the light on. The light and draft-free environment will provide just enough warmth to help the yeast do its thing. Good in the dough. Bad in the gut. Ironic, yes? In 30 minutes or so, the yeast will have doubled. Cut it in half and make two crusts. I use a rolling pin—I stink at hand tossing dough.

To make a tasty gluten-free pizza crust, I recommend you use the King Arthur's gluten-free bread and pizza mix. If you don't have King Arthur in your local stores, you can order it online directly through the company.

CHAPTER 2

Therapy Implementation

When Mia's development slowed down and veered off track, I had no idea where to begin in terms of treatment. I did exactly what, and only what Early Intervention told me to do. In hindsight, that was a mistake. I don't bother beating myself up over this. Let's face it, we'd all be black and blue from head to toe if we self-flagellated every time we made a mistake in trying to help our kids. Lack of knowledge is not stupidity. Lack of money to pay for therapy is not a crime. Both are reality. There are resources available to help you learn more about your options. Then try to prioritize them for your daughter based on efficacy, availability, money, your ability to help implement the therapy, and time requirements.

When working with any sort of therapist, you don't have to be BFFs, but you do have to have a rapport with him or her. That said, you might be taken aback by what appear to be "harsh" techniques in ABA. Don't confuse the therapist's "game face" with personality. Some therapies require tough love. Ask the therapist about his or her style and what reaction(s) you might expect from your child. Knowing that you face a tough challenge lessens the surprise and helps you manage the rough patches.

Paying for It All

Once your daughter is diagnosed as autistic, or anyplace on the spectrum, she is entitled to Medicaid. Google "Medicaid Waiver Programs" in your home state, and you will find organizations that will walk you through the application process, free of charge, and educate you as to just what benefits are included with the waiver programs.

~

When paying for medical expenses, utilize the bucket system:

- **Bucket one:** insurance/Medicaid; if the expense is not covered, then use
- **Bucket Two:** flexible spending accounts; if not eligible (or if they are already used up), then use
- **Bucket Three:** Medical Expense Deduction. If it can be deemed a "good medical expense," save it for tax season.

~

You may also find additional resources through state or local laws that are designed to help children with handicaps (which includes autism, but may not specify as such—for instance, handicapped parking). Research available services provided for your child in your immediate area to obtain maximum benefits, talk to parent "mavens," and ask your local state representatives; they are eager to help their constituents.

How to Build a Treatment Team

Document everything. You will continually call upon all of your autism documents, notes, and records. Organizing your documents will also improve communication between a multidisciplinary health team—not to mention reduce your stress levels!

~

You'll find there is a never-ending pile of application forms needing attention. There is a lot of overlap, so I always have the most commonly asked-for information at hand.

~

Trust your gut when seeking a new treatment provider. You should feel comfortable very early on with your daughter's therapists. Even those with the best reputations do not always mean the best fit for your daughter, you, and your family.

—Lauren Tobing-Puente, PhD, licensed Psychologist,
www.drtobingpuente.com

~

Stay actively involved in your child's treatment. Sit in on some of your child's therapy sessions. Ask questions. Listen to your therapists' feedback. Learn how to reinforce some of the skills that your child is being taught. Offer your own feedback.

—Karen Siff Exkorn, *The Autism Sourcebook*

Applied Behavior Analysis (ABA) Therapy

Applied Behavior Analysis (ABA) therapy is a treatment model that is extremely effective in remediating many of the cognitive-, attention-, and language-based areas of deficit typical to autism. ABA is currently one of the most common interventions, and the core of many educational programs for treating children on the autism spectrum.

—Jenifer Clark, MA, PhD(c), "Applied Behavior Analysis,"
Cutting-Edge Therapies for Autism

~

Applied Behavior Analysis (ABA) is an empirically supported methodology that effectively teaches critical skills to children with autism. An ABA program will typically focus on communication skills, social skills, fine and gross motor skills, and cognitive skills. The basic principles of reinforcement are used to motivate the otherwise unmotivated learner. As the child becomes more connected socially to others, primary reinforcements (such as food) can be replaced by social reinforcers such as praise and tickles. The goals that are set for each child are broken down into their component parts so that the child will be successful. Problem behaviors are either extinguished or replaced. These undesired behaviors can be replaced with alternative behaviors that compete with the unwanted behavior. The positive behavior is heavily reinforced until it replaces the negative behavior so that it is more likely to occur in a given situation.

—Jenifer Clark, MA, PhD(c), MERIT Consulting

~

ABA treatment should begin as early as possible. Children who receive more treatment hours per week (i.e., thirty or more) have better outcomes than those who receive fewer (e.g., fifteen or less); continuing ABA treatment for two or more years will lead to the optimal outcome.

—Dr. Doreen Granpeesheh, Dr. Jonathan Tarbox,
and Dr. Michele Bishop,
"Center for Autism and Related Disorders, Inc. (CARD),"
Cutting-Edge Therapies for Autism

~

Children with ASD might not acquire skills through daily interactions in their home or school environment. To effectively teach children with ASD, tasks are broken down into small, measurable units, and each skill is practiced repeatedly until the child masters the skill. Some skills might serve as building blocks for other more-complex skills (e.g., imitation, attending).

Thus, we might begin working on more-basic skills that allow children to acquire building blocks that prepare the child to learn more advanced skills and learn in a number of different environments. Once a skill is mastered, it is practiced periodically to make sure the child continues to maintain previously mastered skills over time.

—Dr. Tiffany Kodak and Dr. Alison Betz, "Center for
Autism Spectrum Disorders, Munroe-Meyer Institute,"
Cutting-Edge Therapies for Autism

~

The more that parents of children with autism can incorporate sound behavioral practices in a natural way with their autistic child, the better that child's prognosis will be.

—Jenifer Clark, MA, PhD(c), "Applied Behavior Analysis," *Cutting-Edge Therapies for Autism*

~

Cognitive behavioral therapy can be helpful in changing how a person on the more able end of the spectrum thinks about and respond to feelings such as anger, sadness, or anxiety. This can be helpful for girls who are having challenges in dealing with such emotions.

Behavioral Treatment Plans

By Steve Kossor, www.TreatmentPlansThatWorked.com

A behavioral treatment plan should provide all of the information necessary for a conscientious person to deliver the correct treatment procedures, at the correct times, and with sufficient consistency to produce the changes in behavior that are described in the plan—reducing or eliminating undesirable behavior and increasing or improving desired behavior, while providing a means to monitor progress on an ongoing basis that informs the process of treatment.

~

Any behavioral treatment plan should specify the *exact* behavior that is "targeted" for improvement. The plan must say *exactly* what is to be reduced or eliminated. By the same token, the plan must say *exactly* what is to be taught in replacement of the "targeted" behavior. It is rarely helpful to tell a child what *not* to do; you always have to specify what she *should do* as well.

~

A treatment plan should explain *exactly* what the treatment provider should be doing to accomplish the replacement of the "target" behavior. A treatment provider should be able to look at the treatment plan and know precisely which techniques are to be used, how often, and in which circumstances. When terms like "contingency contracting" are used, a glossary of terms that is accessible to the treatment provider is *essential*. How else can the treatment provider know *exactly* what to do?

~

A treatment plan should always contain a simple and easy means of measuring progress from the perspective of the treatment *recipient*, not the treatment provider. Outcome progress measurement should include a "baseline" measure, which is a starting point in the measurement of treatment outcomes that precedes the start of the treatment period. How else will you know how far you've come (or how far you've gone astray) if you don't know where you started?

~

Treatment plans must include a planned stop date, so that the treatment team can prepare to present information to funding authorities prior to that date in order for funding to be continued. Continued funding is necessary and therefore justifiable whenever the child is within the age served by the funding entity, the treatment plan is *working*, but the work has not yet been satisfactorily completed.

Developmental and Relationship Therapies

Floortime: Play with a Purpose. For many kids the most challenging deficits are social and communication delays. These can be addressed through fun parent-child engagements known as floortime. I recommend parents read *Engaging Autism* by Stanley Greenspan and give it a try. Learn more about floortime at the link below; there are instructional videos and information on therapies and how to get trained yourself: www.icdl.com/dirfloor- time/ overview/index.shtml.

~

Other therapies parents can do themselves include Relationship Development Intervention (RDI) and the Ron-Rise program. You will need to be trained by certified consultants in each, but can then implement the programs at home. Check out www.RDIconnect.com and www. AutismTreatmentCenter.org for more information and therapists in your area.

~

Join in their world. If you take the approach pioneered by Stanley Greenspan, you can engage the child by entering their world. Join in their stim or playfully obstruct it in order to engage the child. An example would be to physically block an item or location they want to go. If your child likes to tap a certain area on the floor, sit there. She'll need to get you to move, which requires some level of effort and communication. Think of it as turning into a skid on a slick road in order to gain control of the car.

~

Tasks should be fun. Though it is work to teach your child, the more fun you (and your child's therapists) make it the greater engagement and motivation you will receive from your child.

~

Make the child feel comfortable. They may not appear to be paying attention to you, but they will sense your disposition; make it positive and welcoming. Use high affect and positivity to engage the child.

~

Remember your daughter cannot go from zero to sixty then back down to zero. A typical child can learn to step back and take a breath, but a child with autism can spin herself into her own world; you need to go in and bring her out.

Physical/Occupational Therapy

The earliest forms of physical therapy might include working on skills such as sitting, rolling, crawling, standing, and walking. As the children get older, they might receive physical therapy to address concerns regarding muscle strength, endurance, balance, coordination, motor planning, ball skills, and various forms of locomotion.

—Meghan Collins, "Physical Therapy,"
Cutting-Edge Therapies for Autism

~

Find an occupational therapist: Many children with ASD and sensory integration dysfunction present with low muscle tone and a tendency to rely on end ranges of their joints for stability. This can be illustrated by a child who toe-walks with her back arched, chest out, and her shoulders back. Another example of this is a child who "W"-sits with a rounded back, shoulders forward, and head and neck tilted up. These postures can prevent components of typical movement from occurring that interfere with a child's ability to interact with their world. Both postures prevent side-to-side weight shifting and, in turn, rotation of the trunk. Without rotation, a child's ability to integrate visual, auditory, movement, and spatial information might be significantly impacted.

—Markus Jarrow, "The SMILE Center,"
Cutting-Edge Therapies for Autism

~

Check out occupational therapy—a form of therapy designed to address both sensory needs and motor planning which virtually all ASD kids have. Therapists use a wide variety of tools, including balls, manipulatives, and even Play-Doh to help children learn to tolerate noises, textures, and certain environments. It's also used to address both fine and gross motor skills.

~

No matter how effective the clinician is, he or she might only have an hour or two a week with the child. It is therefore essential that a home program be implemented. This might include simple modifications to the home, adaptations to the child's routines, toys, clothing, etc., as well as specific, scheduled treatment strategies to be carried out in the home and/or school. This is referred to as a sensory diet. This piece is critical in ensuring optimal progress.

—Markus Jarrow, "Occupational Therapy
and Sensory Integration,"
Cutting-Edge Therapies for Autism

~

Sensory issues can often be mistaken for behavioral problems. If a child has vestibular and visual issues, which impact her perception of her position in space, she might have great difficulty sitting upright in a chair without falling from time to time. To avoid falls or embarrassment, she might fidget to better process her body, or get out of her seat often. She, in turn, will present as a child who "won't" stay seated.

—Markus Jarrow, "Occupational Therapy
and Sensory Integration,"
Cutting-Edge Therapies for Autism

～

Play is an open doorway into engaging with students with ASD and the start of a teaching relationship with them.

—Amanda Friedman and Alison Berkley,
"Sensory Gym: Emerge and See,"
Cutting-Edge Therapies for Autism

～

There are two main types of sensory play most children crave: manipulation of self and objects, and release of emotion and energy.

—Amanda Friedman and Alison Berkley,
"Sensory Gym: Emerge and See,"
Cutting-Edge Therapies for Autism

～

Students thrive when learning is interwoven with physical release.

—Amanda Friedman and Alison Berkley,
"Sensory Gym: Emerge and See,"
Cutting-Edge Therapies for Autism

~

A child receiving physical therapy will improve their gross motor function, which is an important aspect of socialization, allowing the child to participate in general play, physical education, or sports. The key to a successful physical therapy session is making the activities during the session motivating for the child. Ultimately kids just want to have fun!

—Meghan Collins, "Physical Therapy,"
Cutting-Edge Therapies for Autism

Speech-Language Therapy

Speech-Language Therapy can provide remediation for the following communication disorders:

- **Language disorder:** impairment of receptive (comprehension), expressive (use of spoken), written, and/or other symbol systems;
- **Speech disorder:** impairment of the articulation of speech sounds, fluency or voice;
- **Pragmatic disorder:** impairment of the ability to use and understand social language (verbal and nonverbal);
- **Hearing disorder:** impairment of the auditory system;
- **Central auditory processing disorder:** impairment of the ability to process, retrieve, and/or organize information through the peripheral and central nervous systems;

- **Prosody disorder:** impairment of the suprasegmentals of speech (intonation, stress).

—Lavinia Pereira and Michelle Solomon,
"Speech-Language Therapy,"
Cutting-Edge Therapies for Autism

~

Children ages zero to three and school-age children might be eligible for speech and language services through the state in which they reside. Government agencies within your state will be able to provide contact information to begin the assessment process, which will determine eligibility for services. School-age children might be evaluated to determine the need for speech-language therapy within the school setting. In addition, licensed therapists in your area can be located by visiting the American Speech-Language-Hearing Association (ASHA) website (www.asha.org), asking your child's doctor, or by contacting local support groups and agencies.

—Lavinia Pereira and Michelle Solomon,
"Speech-Language Therapy,"
Cutting-Edge Therapies for Autism

~

When working with a child on the autism spectrum, it is vital that the surroundings are modified to lessen distractions and provide support for additional needs, such as sensory and attention deficits.

- Decrease visual distractions (little or no decorations)
- Supportive seating
- Facing away from the window
- Good lighting
- Established work area and sensory or "break" area
- Awareness of noises that might be distracting to the child (buzzing of light, air conditioner, heat)
- Toys and materials out of reach and in enclosed cabinets

> —Lavinia Pereira and Michelle Solomon,
> "Speech-Language Therapy,"
> *Cutting-Edge Therapies for Autism*

~

These activities support and encourage communication and interaction:

- Use of routines (daily living activities—dressing, snack time, bedtime routine)
- Use of scripts to learn and practice social scenarios (inviting a peer to play)
- Social stories (address problematic situations by reading stories)
- Repetition of material to foster learning (books, songs, carrier phrases such as "I want")
- Use of cloze sentences ("Birds fly in the (sky)") and fill-ins ("Ready set (go)")
- "Sabotaging" of materials and environment (desired toy out of reach, piece of a toy missing)
- Group therapy (sessions with typical peers to provide modeling of appropriate social behavior)

- Sessions in a natural setting to promote carryover
- Use of technology (computers, handheld game systems) to encourage independent learning and visual feedback
- Establishing a routine to the sessions
- Keep pace of sessions relative to attention span

—Lavinia Pereira and Michelle Solomon,
"Speech-Language Therapy,"
Cutting-Edge Therapies for Autism

~

A naturalistic setting promotes inclusion in "normal" everyday situations, teaches the individual how to interact with others, and allows for more "teachable" moments. Furthermore, when therapy is provided in a natural setting, activities are more purposeful and meaningful, which will increase your child's motivation and desire to participate. For example, an SLP would make learning the labels of food more salient if it is taught and experienced in a kitchen with real food items and engaging activities (cooking, cutting, tasting) versus through the use of pictures and pretend play food in an office or bedroom setting.

—Lavinia Pereira and Michelle Solomon,
"Speech-Language Therapy,"
Cutting-Edge Therapies for Autism

Music Therapy

Many children with autism enjoy and excel in musical activities. Parents can sing with their child, engage in movement and dance, and provide a box of toy instruments. Children with autism who develop an interest in an actual musical instrument can practice their lessons with a parent's encouragement.

—Angie Geisler, "Fun Activity Suggestions
for Parents of Children with Autism,"
www.brighthub.com/education/special/articles/
57559.aspx#ixzz0l0Qc6jnt

CHAPTER 3

Medical and Nutritional Treatment

The following series of tips will give you topline info to help you aid your child from "the inside out." There has been significant coverage in the last two years of something called "the micriobiome" and its connection to brain/gut issues and mental health.

~

"The human microbiome, the collection of trillions of microbes living in and on the human body, is not random, and scientists believe that it plays a role in many basic life processes. As science continues to explore and better understand the identities and activities of the microbial species comprising the human microbiome, microbiologists hope to draw connections between microbiome composition, host genetics, and human health."

—http://academy.asm.org/index.php/
faq-series/5122-humanmicrobiome

~

And from the American Society of Microbiology: "During the first two years of life, infants gradually acquire a microbiome that resembles the typical adult microbiome.

Soon after birth is a unique time when, for example, rare microbes can become established—later they would be out-competed. The recognition that these early years are a crucial time for the establishment of the microbiome has drawn new attention to practices that are fairly recent human introductions—caesarean delivery, formula feeding, and, especially, the use of antibiotics early in life. The long-term impact of different practices on the microbiome is unknown."

"Long-term impact is . . . unknown." That scares me. "We know that pediatric health has changed over the last twenty-five years, as formerly common childhood diseases like chicken pox and, yes, even measles, have been tamped down while chronic conditions like food allergies, asthma, and developmental delays, including Spectrum Disorders" have climbed.

But you don't need a scientific study to know when your child's GI system is not working well. When Mia turned one, I started her on whole milk (I was so excited!) and Cheerios. Within two weeks, she had to have her first suppository. For other kids, diarrhea is the problem. One of the ways to help ameliorate the behaviors of autism is to take an "inside out" approach. That's where biomedical treatment comes into play.

"Biomedical treatment is a systematic approach to treating the underlying issues of autism inside the body. Biomedical treatment is managed by a physician and is individualized to the patient's particular ailments.

Conventional medicine treats the symptoms of autism. Biomedical treatment addresses the root cause.

There are many different biomedical therapies available to treat a child's needs. Many autism symptoms, stims, and behaviors are treatable and can greatly improve through proper treatment."

—http://www.generationrescue.org/
recovery/biomedical-treatment/

~

There are many online resources for credible, practical biomed information. I suggest you go straight to www.tacanow.org and www.generationrescue.org for reams of info, and you can apply for a treatment grant through Generation Rescue. Then talk to other parents on social media and elsewhere. Trust your instincts. No one knows your daughter as well as you do, no matter how many letters he or she has after their name. There is a group called MAPS—Medical Academy of Pediatric Special Needs—dedicated to training doctors who can work with our girls. (http://www.medmaps.org/) Also, check out the list of practitioners on the Generation Rescue site—many are MDs. (http://www.generationrescue.org/resources/find-a-physician/)

For many parents, working through the various biomedical treatments and associated diets is the most challenging component of the battle. It's easy to become overwhelmed with so much information, so it's best to focus on one day and one treatment at a time. And remember: No matter how difficult the day, keep on breathing, because tomorrow is another day. The sun will rise, and who knows what Providence will bring.

How to Find and Choose Your Doctors

Here are some questions to ask when choosing a doctor for your child:

- Approximately how many individuals with autism have you treated? What age range?
- In the event we have a biomedical-related emergency, how will I contact you?
- Do you share an e-mail address, cell-phone number, etc. with your patients?
- Can you collaborate with other specialists we will be dealing with (gastrointestinal, etc.)? Are you willing to collaborate on treatment and testing with my child's pediatrician if he/she is receptive?
- Will you provide a clear plan for supplements and where to purchase them?
- What are the primary medical specialties in which you were originally trained (i.e., pediatrics, family medicine)? What is now the primary focus of your practice? If you are not an MD or DO, in what field(s) are you licensed?
- Do you sell proprietary nutritional supplements or have a sales agreement with supplement suppliers? Do you sell supplements at cost?
- Do you bill for laboratory tests done by commercial laboratories? how do you break down the fees?

—Autism Research Institute,
www.autism.com/pro_questions.asp

~

At the link below you can find a list of physicians and licensed health care professionals is provided as a resource. Each physician is trained in autism treatments, parent recommended and vetted by Generation Rescue.

—http://www.generationrescue.org/ resources/find-a-physician/

~

You will want to include your child's pediatrician in the overall treatment strategy (biomedical, educational, therapies, etc.). It is imperative that the pediatrician allows time for you to discuss concerns, and for them to devote the time to work with you in addressing those concerns.

Diet. Try it!

You have probably heard of "the diet." THAT diet. (Said like a true four letter word.) This usually means the gluten-free/casein-free diet, the grandpappy of "Oh dear Lord how will I ever feed my daughter" dietary interventions for autism. It took me over a year to work up the gumption to get my daughters onto the diet. A. Year. Their first GF/CF breakfast was potato chips and orange juice. So don't beat yourself up if your first reaction is "Heck no!" You can start the diet and see results that range from "not-so-much" to profoundly life changing.

~

The *Talk about Curing Autism* website has, hands-down, the best information on how to start several autism friendly diets, how to stay on the diet, pay for the diet, and how to explain to Grandma that her butter cookie recipe is no longer an option without being disinherited. Don't laugh—family and friends are often roadblocks to success and can sabotage your hard work and compromise your daughter's progress.

—https://www.tacanow.org/tag/gfcf/

~

If you begin to suspect a particular food item might be impacting behavior, test. Give your daughter two weeks away from the item and observe the results. It will be another clue for your medical team. Don't forget to remind folks at school about this, and other food restrictions.

~

You wouldn't let your typical child live on a diet of Goldfish crackers and skittles. Your child with autism is no different.

—Judith Chinitz, MS, MS, CNC, author of *We Band of Mothers*

~

As a group, children with autism have notoriously poor nutrition coupled with vitamin and mineral deficiencies. This may be due, in part, to extreme eating habits (they are notoriously picky). Deficiencies are also likely due to the abovementioned tendency toward malabsorption. This is why physicians who specialize in

the biomedical treatment of autism start out by addressing
malabsorption issues, adding digestive enzymes to the diet,
eliminating problematic foods (usually including gluten
and casein), stabilizing the condition of the gastrointestinal
tract by removing allergens and harmful organisms,
and introducing nutrients not being properly absorbed
and utilized by the body. This approach has resulted in
significant improvement in cognitive function, and in some
cases, a full recovery from many of the symptoms of autism,
if not the underlying disorder.

~

This approach can be challenging for parents. Changes in
diet and supplementation are not usually expensive, but
can be hard to implement. There are no guarantees, but
thousands of parents will tell you that it is worth the effort.
Changes in behavior, improvements in bowel function,
increased language, and decreased self-stimulation are
common responses to biomedical interventions. But if you're
going to do it, commit to doing it fully—halfway measures
are unlikely to bring about improvement.

~

Identify the Pre-Diet Diet: Make a list of all the foods
your child likes and eats. What do they have in common?
Perhaps they are all starchy, sweet, salty, dairy-based, or
wheat-based. Perhaps they are all the same types of foods. A
child eating ice cream, bananas, grapes, chocolate pudding,
sweetened yogurt, apple juice, and ketchup is not eating

a varied diet—he is eating milk and sugar. A child who only eats bagels, crackers, cereal, pretzels, and waffles is not eating a varied diet; he is mostly eating one food: wheat. Foods that are craved are highly suspect, especially dairy- and wheat-based foods. Next, make a list of your child's physical symptoms. Does he get rashes? Does he get red cheeks or red ears after meals? Is his stomach bloated? Does he have diarrhea or constipation? Is he insensitive to pain? Note how these symptoms are associated with food; for example, does your child get red cheeks shortly after eating a particular food? Are bowel problems associated with any particular types of food? Are his behaviors worse at certain times of day, before or after meals?

~

Commit to a three-month trial of dietary intervention. Join an online support group such as the one at www.gfcfdiet. com. Choose a date, planning a day or two's meals at a time.

~

Start a food diary—this will turn out to be an important tool and should not be overlooked. Get a spiral pad or notebook and list each food your child eats on the left side of the page. On the right side of the page, list any changes you observe. Make a note of things like aggression, crying, whining, red ears, itchiness, bowel changes, or sleep problems.

~

It is common to see crankiness, regression, or withdrawal symptoms during these first few days. Stay the course, and let your child know that you mean business.

~

Keep it simple: Instead of providing homemade or commercially available chicken nuggets, teach your children to eat plain chicken that has been baked or broiled. Cut the chicken into child-friendly strips and serve with a simple dipping sauce that you can make from scratch, quickly and cheaply. Teach your children to eat fruits and vegetables that are raw or gently steamed, again, using a simple sauce at first if they won't even try them plain, or blending them into pasta sauce or soup.

~

For those who are willing to learn to follow some simple recipes at home, dietary intervention shouldn't increase your family's food bill by very much. In fact, it may save you quite a bit of money, since you are far more likely to pack healthy, safe foods before leaving the house, and far less likely to grab a meal at a fast-food restaurant.

~

Get support: Compile a few articles on diet that you can give family members, teachers, and other caregivers. Tell them what you are doing, and why. Ask for their support.

~

Remember: Just because the child does not test positive for wheat and dairy allergy does not mean that these foods are tolerated.

~

Sometimes changing the diet can lead to striking results within a short period of time. Younger children who are drinking large quantities of milk or eating primarily dairy- or wheat-based foods might exhibit changes within a week. But for most, the change won't be apparent until a few weeks later—often after accidental ingestion, when there is a noticeable regression. You might notice changes within a few days, but if not, be patient.

~

Most people get the hang of the diet in a week or two, and many good substitutes are now available for traditional wheat products. There are commercially available gluten-free breads at many supermarkets and at all health-food stores. Crackers without wheat or gluten are also widely available, made from grains, rice, and even nuts. If your child likes pasta, there are many excellent gluten-free alternatives; they come in different shapes and sizes and can be used in any recipe. Gluten-free baking, once you get the hang of it, is an economical way to prepare your family's favorite baked goods at home.

~

If you're thinking, "But the only things my picky eater is willing to eat are gluten- and casein-based," you're not alone. In fact, these children are the likeliest responders. Some parents say, "I can't possibly consult a nutritionist or dietitian—my child is a picky eater." Professionals are trained to address picky eating—they don't often hear from parents of children who happily eat a wide array of healthy lean meats, fruits, and vegetables.

~

Getting Enough Calcium with the GF/CF Diet:

- Green vegetables such as kale, collards, and bok choy are excellent sources of calcium, with the added benefit of being low in oxalates (spinach, though high in calcium, should be avoided if oxalates are a problem).
- Certain fish, like salmon and perch, are also good sources of calcium, but take care to buy fish that is not high in mercury or other environmental toxins (the smaller ones).
- A mere tablespoon of molasses contains 172 mg of calcium (as well as iron), so if yeast is not a big problem, it is a good choice for sweetening baked goods.
- Some nuts, beans, and seeds (like sesame seeds) are rich in calcium, but they should be ground for best absorption.
- Finally, if a child will not eat enough nondairy sources of calcium, there are many good supplements available. Because vitamin D is required to properly absorb calcium, a good supplement will contain both.

~

To eliminate the chance of ingesting toxins via food, avoid toxic fish, especially those who are the larger longer-living species such as swordfish, which wind up absorbing more of the mercury in the ocean. Others in the group include tilefish and marlin and shark. Check out the following site from the Natural Resources Defense Council for a more detailed list of fish with the most, and least mercury: www.nrdc.org/health/effects/mercury/guide.asp.

~

Keep in mind that "nondairy" does not mean milk-free. It is a term the dairy industry invented to indicate less than 0.5 percent milk by weight, which could mean fully as much casein as whole milk.

~

While it might be unrealistic to expect your entire family to take this novel dietary path, the benefits of introducing everyone to more whole foods should be obvious. We began the GF/CF (gluten-free, casein-free) diet as a family so that [our daughter] wouldn't feel singled out or deprived.

—Julie A. Buckley, MD, *Healing Our Autistic Children*

~

Find a biomedical "maven," someone already ahead of you on the learning curve. This could be another parent you know, someone from a parent social group, or your child's school. If you cannot find someone nearby that you trust, you can contact organizations such as the National Autism

Association (NAA), Talk About Curing Autism (TACA), or Generation Rescue (GR). All have lists of parents who are biomedical mavens and donate their time to talk to parents who are new to the approach. Check out the NAA and GR sites. NAA calls their mavens "Naavigators" and GR calls them "Rescue Angels."

~

Keep a diary, including what your child takes and ultimately eats, along with results such as hyperactivity level, bowel movements, stimming, and any tantrums.

~

From my experience, the behavioral and cognitive symptoms of many ASD children can be noticeably improved with proper biomedical treatments. Sometimes the improvement is dramatic enough for a child to lose his or her ASD diagnosis.

—Jaquelyn McCandless, *Children with Starving Brains*

~

Before starting down this road, remember that most recoveries and improvements have taken considerable time. In many cases your child has been "sick" for a while, and there is no quick fix. Think of biomedical therapy as a marathon that will take considerable time and perseverance, so you need to pace yourself. And, most important, a marathon is much more mental than physical; mental strength is the key. There is no magic bullet.

~

Don't count on yourself to notice and remember progress—or lack thereof—keep careful notes. You'll often find yourself thinking, "Wow—I had forgotten that she used to do that."

~

Younger kids may respond quicker, but do not give up if they don't. Also, kids are never too old to start. Plus, you never know what treatments will become available; there are new therapies to try every year. Keep breathing and moving forward!

~

Do your own research, and do not rely solely on your doctor to know all. You as a parent are the key advocate for your child, and you need to be active in the treatment process. Learn all there is to know about autism, and share it with the doctor(s). This education will help you understand the complex treatment process and keep you on task during difficult periods. You might have a great doctor, but no one cares as much as you do about the health of your child.

~

Be aggressive early. You have the best chance of helping your child when they are very young, so don't put off treatments. You don't ever want to look back and say, "if only . . ."

—Judith Chinitz, MS, MS, CNC, author of *We Band of Mothers*

~

When it comes to treatment for your child: If it can't hurt, and it could help, then do it. If it *can* hurt, then weigh the possible risks against the possible rewards. If the latter is heavier, then do it.

—Judith Chinitz, MS, MS, CNC, author of *We Band of Mothers*

~

The best laboratory is your child (according to Dr. Sidney Baker). The only way to really know if a treatment is going to work is to try it. We don't have the lab testing to predict individual reactions.

—Judith Chinitz, MS, MS, CNC, author of *We Band of Mothers*

~

Become an educated consumer; familiarize yourself with PubMed, the government's database of published research (www.ncbi.nlm.nih.gov/sites/pubmed). When considering a possible treatment, search PubMed first and weigh the evidence.

~

When beginning biomedical therapies, it's best not to begin everything at once. Try to phase things in over the course of weeks and months so that you can determine what might and might not be working. If you start too much at once, you will not know what is working or what could be causing problems.

~

Children already affected by autism can and do recover or significantly improve when a combination of biomedical and behavioral/educational therapies are employed. Doreen Granpeesheh, PhD, BCBA-D, founder and executive director of the Center for Autism and Related Disorders, agrees: "While behavioral/educational and biomedical practitioners have individually helped provide successful treatment models for autism, working together, these interventions have led to the best possibilities for successful outcome."

—Teri Arranga, "Afterword,"
Cutting-Edge Therapies for Autism

~

Keep some sort of journal of therapies and treatments along with reactions. We have a spreadsheet that you can download to help you with this. Update this (or a similar log) daily, and over time, you will be able to see what is working, and share this information with your doctor and therapists. Visit www.skyhorsepublishing.com/Therapy_logbook.xls.

~

Continue to keep good records of the improvements you see in your child's behaviors, as they are probably the most significant measure of any therapy's effectiveness.

—Julie A. Buckley, MD, *Healing Our Autistic Children*

~

Two steps forward, one step back—most children with autism have progress followed by plateau or regression; it's best to look for the overall trend.

~

When giving supplements, it's best to teach your daughter to take pills/capsules, but in the interim, utilize liquids, powders, and chewables as available (most come in multiple formulations). Anything in a capsule can be mixed into food or drink.

~

What if your kid doesn't swallow pills? There are two important keys to success with this, the roux and the meat injector! Empty all your capsules into a small cup with highish sides (I use a 3 oz. Tupperware container), add any additional powders. Then add a tiny bit of liquid (I use filtered water or liquid molybdenum, depending on whether it is morning or evening)—just enough to make a roux (or thick paste), if you add too much liquid, the powders will clump and you will have a mess. Stir it thoroughly so it has an even consistency then add more water to almost fill the cup. Next comes the meat injector! Use a meat injector instead of a syringe (a syringe is at most 2T, a meat injector holds much more liquid)—you can purchase one at Bed Bath and Beyond or any store that carries cooking tools. Remove the needle, suck up the supplement stew and squirt it into your child's mouth.

—Peggy Lowery Becker, mom of an 11-year-old ASD boy

~

Watch the use of digestive enzymes, as they will break down pro-biotics; be sure to allow at least an hour between the two.

~

Likewise, zinc could interfere with the absorption of other minerals and some vitamins; give zinc a window of an hour or two.

~

If using powders or breaking open caps, you can mix into foods or try making a smoothie. It's a good way to get some nice antioxidant berries and other good stuff down with the supps at the same time.

~

Some prescribed meds may only be available compounded, or they are easier to use in a compound form. Just remember that if you have Medicaid for your daughter, the compounding pharmacy has to be in your home state, or else Medicaid will not cover it (it's a state program).

~

Activated charcoal. AC lessens the die-offs associated with anti-fungal treatments and other antioxidant products. AC also serves to help with any GI disturbances, use it yourself and see! Just remember to give two hours before or after other meds/supplements, as it will not discriminate in what is absorbs and removes.

~

Home remedies: Epsom salt baths act as a natural detoxifier and also aid in constipation and help calming! The one occasional negative can be dry skin; if your child experiences dry skin, just add some baking soda to the mix.

~

When dealing with constipation, remember one good "cleaning" is not all it takes. In most cases it took your child years to develop the condition, you need to get her regular for months to shrink the colon back to size!

~

For handling constipation there are a number of reliable and safe non-medical alternatives including supplementing magnesium (consult a physician for dosage), aloe juice (pour a little into the morning OJ) and Fruit-Eze, which is a prune, raisin, and date jam. If your child doesn't like the taste you can cover with something like peanut butter or syrup.

The Metabolic System

Many of the metabolic abnormalities and susceptibilities that we commonly see in autism can be explained after examining the effects of acquired or inherited abnormalities in methylation and detoxification pathways. It's interesting to note that nutritional supplements associated with an improvement in autistic symptoms, either anecdotally or in the medical literature, happen to support normal function of these pathways. These include folinic acid, DMG, TMG, methylcobalamin, zinc, vitamin B6 (or P5P), digestive enzymes containing DPP-IV, GSH, cysteine (as N-acetyl cysteine), sulfate, and metallothionein-promoting amino acids.

—Reprinted by permission of the publisher. From Bryan Jepson, M.D., and Jane Johnson, *Changing the Course of Autism: A Scientific Approach for Parents and Physicians*, Boulder, CO: Sentient Publications. Copyright © 2007 by Bryan Jepson and Jane Johnson. All rights reserved.

~

Though methyl-B12 shots are initially feared by most parents, they soon learn that the shots are nearly painless, easy to administer, and give the greatest number of clinical responses when compared to oral, nasal, or transdermal routes of administration.

—Dr. James Neubrander, "Methyl–B12: Myth or Masterpiece," *Cutting-Edge Therapies for Autism*

~

For children with autism, the results of transmethylation are increased language, focus and attention, awareness, cognition, independence, socialization and interactive play, appropriate emotional responses, affection, eye contact, and improvements in gross and fine motor skills.

—Dr. James Neubrander, "Methyl–B12: Myth or Masterpiece,"
Cutting-Edge Therapies for Autism

~

The following is adapted from Dr. Richard E. Frye, "Mitochondrial Dysfunction," *Cutting-Edge Therapies for Autism*:

- Individuals with mitochondrial dysfunction should avoid physiological stressors.
- Patients should avoid fasting, extreme cold or heat, sleep deprivation, dehydration, and illness.
- If an individual with mitochondrial dysfunction becomes sick, there should be aggressive control of fever and hydration. During illness an individual with mitochondrial dysfunction should be closely monitored and provided intravenous hydration with carbohydrates if necessary.
- Certain drugs and environmental toxins which depress mitochondrial function should be avoided. Common toxins that inhibit mitochondrial function include heavy metals, insecticides, cigarette smoke, and monosodium glutamate. common drugs that inhibit mitochondrial function include acetaminophen, nonsteroidal anti–inflammatory drugs, alcohol, some antipsychotic, antidepressant, anticonvulsant, antidiabetic, antihyperlipidemic, antibiotic, and anesthetic drugs.

- For some patients an overnight fast can be enough to destabilize mitochondrial function.
- Such patients can be treated with complex carbohydrates such as corn starch before bedtime. Some can be awakened in the middle of the night for a snack, while others might require a feeding tube to receive feeding overnight.
- Other patients respond to high-fat diets such as the ketogenic diet.
- Some patients respond to medium chain triglyceride oil supplementation, since these fats do not require carnitine to be transported into the mitochondria.
- Most vitamins are well tolerated, even at high doses. some children with autism might have behavioral side effects from some vitamins. Thus, it is important to start vitamins one at a time, so that any side effects can be linked to a particular vitamin.
- Levocarnitine is linked to behavioral disturbances, especially in children with fatty acid abnormalities.
- Pyridoxine has been suggested to result in peripheral neuropathy at high doses.
- Children should be carefully monitored when the ketogenic diet is started, as the diet can worsen the metabolic acidosis associated with mitochondrial dysfunction.

The Immune System

There's a great body of evidence in the literature documenting immune dysregulation in autistic children leaving them prone to infection, chronic inflammation, and autoimmune reactions; it can affect any organ system, but the brain and the GI tract seem to be the worst hit. These immune system issues haven't been traced to a single underlying abnormality, and aren't always consistent among children on the autism spectrum. Just as there are subgroups based on behavioral characteristics, there appear to be subgroups within the autism spectrum related to the type and severity of immune abnormalities.

> —Reprinted by permission of the publisher. From Bryan Jepson, MD, and Jane Johnson, *Changing the Course of Autism: A Scientific Approach for Parents and Physicians*, Boulder, CO: Sentient Publications. Copyright © 2007 by Bryan Jepson and Jane Johnson. All rights reserved.

~

Autistic children have abnormal immune function, including low natural killer cell function and a TH1/TH2 imbalance. This means that affected children are much more likely to develop allergies and antibodies and a lot less able to kill off infections. They have chronic inflammation and autoimmune reactions. Many of them have eczema, chronic runny noses, ear infections—they seem to be sick all the time. I also see kids on the other end of the spectrum who never get sick. Even though the rest of the family is sick, they're fine. This suggests a hyper-immune state. These are the kids who are more likely to have autoantibodies. The body attacks itself because the immune system is on hyperdrive.

> —Bryan Jepson, MD, Medical Director, Thoughtful House Center for Children

~

Children might acquire viral infections at birth, in the perinatal period and beyond. signs of viral infections in children with autism, due to increased TH2 response and immune suppression, are often not the usual signs of acute infection: nasal congestion, fever, cough, and/or nausea and vomiting. Chronic viral infections cause other symptoms: low endurance, rashes that come and go, and prolonged or intermittent low-grade fever. The children tire easily, have chronic congestion after allergy elimination, and are irritable.

—Dr. Mary Megson, "Viruses and Autism,"
Cutting-Edge Therapies for Autism

The Gastrointestinal System

Children with autism frequently have gastrointestinal problems, particularly constipation and diarrhea. When a child has GI symptoms, we generally find inflammation somewhere along the GI tract, but particularly in the terminal ileum, on endoscopy as well as biopsy. Many autistic children have evidence of abnormal intestinal permeability, or what we call "leaky gut." We continually find inflammatory bowel disease that is different from Crohn's disease and ulcerative colitis.

—Bryan Jepson, MD, Medical Director,
Thoughtful House Center for Children

~

Undiagnosed abdominal issues are the cause of many of the behavior symptoms of autism. If you imagine yourself as a non-verbal or poorly communicative individual who has chronic or intermittent abdominal pain, a lot of your behaviors are going to look pretty autistic. One example is abnormal posturing. We see some children go to great lengths to put pressure on their lower abdomen. They'll lie on the corner of a table or the arm of a sofa for hours. This was once considered an autistic behavior, but we now know that it's done exclusively to ease pain. What we've learned is that when you treat the abdominal symptoms, a lot of what were considered autistic behaviors disappear if your child has frequent nighttime awakenings and/or wettings, they should have a full GI workup; nighttime awakenings can mean reflux, and wettings can mean allergies.

~

The presence of chronic (i.e., long-standing) GI symptoms demands medical evaluation. The fact that the child has autism is merely an interesting sidebar item. The symptoms typically consist of any (or all) of the following:

- Abdominal pain
- Diarrhea (defined as unformed stool that does not hold its own shape but rather conforms to the shape of the container/nappy/diaper that it is in)
- Constipation (defined as infrequent passage of stool of any consistency or passage of overly hard stools regardless of frequency)
- Soft-stool constipation

- Painful passage of unformed stool
- Rectal prolapse
- Failure to maintain normal growth
- Regurgitation
- Rumination
- Abdominal distention
- Food avoidance

—Dr. Arthur Krigsman, "Gastrointestinal Disease:
Emerging Consensus,"
Cutting-Edge Therapies for Autism

~

Parents, physicians, and therapists must realize that difficult-to-treat ASD behaviors or behaviors that have not been responsive to standard behavioral interventions might be the sole manifestation of a GI diagnosis. This means that unprovoked aggression, violent behavior, and irritability might have an underlying GI cause, and this must be taken into consideration prior to the reflexive desire to begin a psychotropic drug such as risperidone (despite its FDA approval for the treatment of autism).

—Dr. Arthur Krigsman, "Gastrointestinal Disease:
Emerging Consensus,"
Cutting-Edge Therapies for Autism

~

Gastroesophageal reflux disease, gastritis/gastric ulcer, and constipation are just three examples of GI diagnoses that are known to cause behavioral symptoms. In addition, poor focus and an inability to make significant academic or communicative progress despite intensive interventions might indicate the presence of treatable bowel disease that, once treated, can significantly improve the child's degree of disability.

> —Dr. Arthur Krigsman, "Gastrointestinal Disease:
> Emerging Consensus,"
> *Cutting-Edge Therapies for Autism*

~

Treatment of GI disease should follow established treatment protocols for the particular diagnosis.

> —Dr. Arthur Krigsman, "Gastrointestinal Disease:
> Emerging Consensus,"
> *Cutting-Edge Therapies or Autism*

~

GI diagnoses unique to ASD require further study to determine best treatment practices.

> —Dr. Arthur Krigsman, "Gastrointestinal Disease:
> Emerging Consensus,"
> *Cutting-Edge Therapies for Autism*

~

Many doctors have noted that children with autism often have gut problems. Inflammation can be a major problem. Tissues that are inflamed are damaged. Damaged cells don't produce enzymes; therefore, many children with autism might present with deficiencies in some enzymes until the gut is healed and operating normally. Malabsorption might present as well. Food intolerance and outright food allergies might also manifest in these children.

—Dr. Devin Houston, "Enzymes for Digestive Support in Autism," *Cutting-Edge Therapies for Autism*

~

Enzymes might be helpful in other ways for those with autism. Keeping the gut free of undigested material prevents putrefaction that might lead to pathogenic bacterial blooms and yeast problems.

—Dr. Devin Houston, "Enzymes for Digestive Support in Autism," *Cutting-Edge Therapies for Autism*

~

Gas and bloating might be minimized by using carbohydrase enzymes such as lactase and alpha-galactosidase. Some vegetables contain carbohydrates such as stachyose and raffinose that are difficult for humans to digest. The human gut lacks the enzymes to degrade carbohydrates that become a food source for gas- producing bacteria. Alpha-galactosidase enzyme supplements can make up for the deficiency and ease the bloating. Chronic diarrhea might also be helped through the addition of enzymes such as amylase and glucoamylase that degrade starchy foods.

—Dr. Devin Houston, "Enzymes for
Digestive Support in Autism,"
Cutting-Edge Therapies for Autism

~

Give probiotics and prebiotics after a meal to maximize absorption, as stomach acid is then otherwise engaged.

~

The tips below are medical in nature, and I'll let them stand on their own. Finding specialists you trust and a pediatrician who can help you coordinate care is very difficult. How to say this nicely . . . wait! I'm Kim, I don't have to say anything nicely. Some doctors are just plain asses when it comes to our daughters. Often our girls fall outside the norms in terms their ability to tolerate testing, sit for or during an appointment, explain their aches, pains, symptoms. They also fall outside of the "norms" for autism. Plus, you and I might enter the office loaded for bear so to speak. As exhaustion and frustration take their toll. My daughters and I have stymied even the best intentioned doctors. Most testing comes back "normal," and we're sitting at square one. Normal is a dirty word as far as I'm concerned.

Talk to other parents about which docs are having success with the medical issues of autism. Ask to schedule a double appointment block and bring someone who can sit with your child in the waiting area while you talk to the physician alone. Write notes. Bring notes. If your insurance company offers a care coordinator, get one and develop a relationship. My girls were on Medicaid and we got out-of-state treatment with a specialist covered thanks to a diligent care coordinator who (drumroll please) had a son with autism. Plus $.45 a mile for the 1200 mile roundtrip to see him because our case manager had a brain and a heart.

Seizures

The following tips are from Dr. Richard E. Frye, "Antiepileptic Medications," *Cutting-Edge Therapies for Autism*:

- **Seizure Syndromes:** Individuals with epilepsy related to a specific epilepsy syndrome, such as tuberous sclerosis, should be treated with AEDs that are effective for treating the specific underlying epilepsy syndrome.

- **Emergency Seizure Treatment:** In many cases, rectal diazepam is very effective to treat prolonged seizure activity and may be prescribed to individuals with epilepsy or seizures that are at risk for such a prolonged seizure.

- **Epileptic Encephalopathy:** AEDs have been more extensively studied for the classically recognized epileptic encephalopathies, specifically Landau-Kleffner syndrome and electrical status epilepticus during slow-wave sleep, than the less well-characterized syndromes such as subclinical electrical discharges. In general, the same medications appear to be just as effective for all the epileptic encephalopathies. Valproate has efficacy in some cases and may be the initial treatment choice. Occasionally, oxcarbazepine may be helpful for very focal electrical discharges. Immunomodulatory treatments, specifically steroids and intravenous immunoglobulin, may also be helpful adjunctive treatments for these syndromes. For electrical status epilepticus during slow-wave sleep, diazepam prior to sleep has also been used.

- **Behavior and Mood Regulation:** Valproate and lamotrigine are particularly effective in mood regulation, while topiramate appears to be effective for reducing impulsivity and aggressive behavior.

- **Migraine Headaches:** Valproate, gabapentin, and topiramate have been very effective in treating migraine headaches, with topiramate being particularly effective.

- **Periodic Leg Movements during Sleep:** Gabapentin can be useful for treating period leg movements during sleep, especially if there is trouble with sleep initiation.

~

For the approximately one in five children with autism who suffer some sort of seizure disorder, it is important to note that marijuana is an excellent anticonvulsant, and was widely used as such in the last part of the nineteenth century and the early decades of the twentieth. Inhalation is not an option for children who suffer from autism; for these patients, the best route for administration is oral, in the form of cookies, brownies, tea, etc. Marijuana cookbooks are now available from which a variety of edibles that appeal to children can be found. With ingestion, the therapeutic effects will not appear before one and a half to two hours, but the advantage is that they last for many hours.

> —Dr. Lester Grinspoon, "Medicinal Marijuana: A Novel Approach to the Symptomatic Treatment of Autism," *Cutting-Edge Therapies for Autism*

~

Well if that tip doesn't cry out for a brownie recipe, I don't know which one does! Buy the King Arthur Flour GF brownie mix and follow the directions. Ta-da! Make sure you add chocolate chips to the top and walnuts if your daughter can tolerate nuts. King Arthur Flour is headquartered in my neighboring state to the north, Vermont. I can find the mixes in many grocery store chains here. However, for the best selection, at the best price, and for those of you who might not have access to this brand nearby, I recommend ordering directly online. Get onto their mailing list and you'll get alerts for savings and free shipping. I love having a cabinet full of blue and white boxes so that I can bake GF/CF anytime (www.kingarthurflour.com). There are other brands of boxed GF brownie mixes, including Betty Crocker and Bob's Red Mill. They all produce a moist, chewy brownie that your entire family will enjoy.

To Medicate or Not to Medicate?

You might be surprised to learn that while I have three daughters with autism, we have taken only one "prescription" medication—by which I mean a medicine prescribed by an allopathic doctor and available at CVS or Walgreens. That was a seizure med when Mia was a youngster. My personal decision for my girls was to try to treat their behaviors and other autism related issues with biomedical treatments, food, and a whole lot of prayers. Not every parent takes this route, and many kids benefit from careful medication with a patient and resourceful physician. Trust your instinct and choose the path you think is best for your girl. When talking about medical choices, I usually tell parents, "Which decision will help you sleep at night?" I'll let the experts talk to you about meds.

~

Medication can be used for the short term. Once your child starts a med, you aren't necessarily committing him to years of treatment. If you see positive results, your child can continue to take it for several months to a year, and then he can be weaned off it to see if it is still needed. Often a child matures or responds to all of his other therapies to the point that medication is no longer needed.

—Robert Sears, *The Autism Book*

~

71

Before accepting a drug prescription, ask a lot of questions, especially ones, such as: Are there any possible side effects? Will his sleep be affected? What is in the actual drug? How exactly does it work on my child's mind? Also ask about the success/non-success rate, as this is usually important when it comes to letting you know how effective the drug may be for your child's particular needs. Medications are not something to be treated lightly.

~

Signs that would alert you to the need for medication management include:

- Your child's safety is being questioned
- Increased episodes of physical aggression toward self and others
- Episodes of physical or verbal aggression are prolonged and not responsive to other intervention techniques
- Uncontrolled temper tantrums
- Fear that your child will hurt you or other members of your family or support team
- Increase in repetitive or stereotypic behaviors despite other interventions being in place
- Increase in anxiety, impulsivity, and inattention despite other interventions being in place

—Dr. Mark Freilich, "Pharmaceutical Medication Management: The Why, When, and What," *Cutting-Edge Therapies for Autism*

Medical and Nutritional Treatment

~

Manifestations that may be helped by various
pharmacologic agents include:

- Attention/distractibility/focus
- Repetitive/stereotypic behaviors
- Depression
- Anxiety
- Severe irritability
- Aggression/self-injurious behaviors
- Mood stabilization

> —Dr. Mark Freilich, "Pharmaceutical Medication
> Management: The Why, When, and What,"
> *Cutting-Edge Therapies for Autism*

~

Antipsychotic drugs and mood stabilizers might help
autistic patients who repeatedly injure themselves.

> —Dr. Lester Grinspoon, "Medicinal Marijuana: A Novel
> Approach to the Symptomatic Treatment of Autism,"
> *Cutting-Edge Therapies for Autism*

~

Anticonvulsants might be useful in suppressing explosive
rage and calming severe anxiety.

> —Dr. Lester Grinspoon, "Medicinal Marijuana: A Novel
> Approach to the Symptomatic Treatment of Autism,"
> *Cutting-Edge Therapies for Autism*

~

The psychoactive medications that are most often used to treat autism are in the following major categories:

- Antidepressants
- Atypical antipsychotics (or neuroleptics)
- Anticonvulsants
- Stimulants (or ADHD medications)
- Anti-opioids
- Miscellaneous medications

—Kenneth Bock, MD, *Healing the New Childhood Epidemics*

~

The Autism Research Institute has surveyed more than 27,000 parents since 1967; often-prescribed meds like Risperdal, Ritalin, and Prozac are by no means the most successful treatments. Before choosing psychotropic meds that often have unpleasant side effects, consider dietary intervention. Read ARI's survey: http://autism.com/pdf/providers/Parentratings2009.pdf, and consider biomedical treatment. Make sure all educational therapies are appropriately implemented.

~

Symptoms such as aggression and self-injurious behavior are often responses to pain. Before assuming a psychological genesis, be 100 percent certain that your child is not in pain. In particular, stomach pain and/or gastroesophageal reflux should be ruled out.

~

Today there are many new drug treatments that can be
really helpful to people with autism. These medications
are especially useful for problems that occur after puberty.
Unfortunately, many medical professionals do not know
how to prescribe them properly.

—Temple Grandin, PhD, *Thinking in Pictures*

~

Medication as a first line of action may allow the child
to be- come more available to the positive effects of the
various other treatment approaches that have been deemed
appropriate. This can lead to a reduction in or the eventual
elimination of medication.

—Dr. Mark Freilich, "Pharmaceutical Medication
Management: The Why, When, and What,"
Cutting-Edge Therapies for Autism

~

If you choose to medicate, keep in mind that people
with autism are often exquisitely sensitive to medication.
Sometimes a surprisingly small dose can be effective. Be
wary of professionals who don't understand this, and use a
one-size-fits-all approach.

~

The process of determining the appropriate medication
and the appropriate dosage cannot be completed

overnight. The process will, at first, require weekly office visits (or at least weekly telephone communication) with the prescribing physician. If, at any point before finding the "optimal" dosage, the physician hands you a prescription and tells you that the plan is to administer the medication and return in a month's time, please consider another medication manager.

—Dr. Mark Freilich, "Pharmaceutical Medication Management: The Why, When, and What," *Cutting-Edge Therapies for Autism*

Preparing for that Inevitable Emergency Room Visit

Having a first aid kit at home is of absolute necessity, as is knowing how to use it! Take a class in first aid at your local firehouse or medical facility and you may be able to save a visit to the doctor or other such facility that can be traumatic for our kids.

～

To adjust to minor cuts and scrapes, let your child play wear a band-aid now and then so the actual need is no big deal. Let them practice on you. Wear a band-aid yourself, or if there is a chronic issue try to mimic what they will have deal with so that they can become a bit more comfortable with the process.

～

Thank you to fellow Skyhorse author Susan K. Delaine for this recipe from her cookbook.

HAMBURGER OR CHEESEBURGER PIE

FILLING INGREDIENTS
½ pound ground beef or turkey
1 small onion, chopped
½ cup canned or frozen corn, drained
½ cup peeled, frozen carrot slices (optional)
¼ cup tomato sauce
¼ cup water
½ teaspoon crushed thyme
Salt and pepper to taste
Daiya Cheddar Shreds for cheeseburger (optional)

TOPPING INGREDIENTS (½ batch of *The Autism Cookbook* cornbread batter)
1 cup organic cornmeal
1 tablespoon light buckwheat flour
2 teaspoons aluminum-free baking powder
¼ teaspoon salt
2 tablespoons evaporated cane juice
¼ cup unsweetened applesauce
¼ cup corn oil, safflower oil, or light olive oil
½ cup water

Preheat oven to 400°F. Brown the meat in a medium skillet and drain the fat. Add onion, corn and carrots. Cook over low heat until onion is soft, stirring frequently. Remove from heat and add tomato sauce and water. Stir until blended. Add thyme, and add the salt and pepper to taste. Pour the meat into a 9x9 baking dish and spread evenly. For a cheeseburger variation, spread a generous amount of Daiya Cheddar shreds evenly over the meat. Set aside.

Meanwhile, prepare cornbread topping. In a medium bowl, combine dry ingredients and stir. Add wet ingredients and stir until blended. Pour the batter over the meat and spread evenly with a rubber spatula. Bake 25–30 minutes, or until the cornbread appears light brown and crusty around the edges.

Let stand 15 minutes before serving.

From *The Autism Cookbook: 101 Gluten-Free and Dairy-Free Recipes*, by Susan K. Delaine ©2010 Skyhorse Publishing.

The Dentist

Mia, Gianna, and Bella's grandfather (my Dad) was an orthodontist. I grew up hearing, "Open, bite," at the dinner table during an impromptu examination of my teeth. For my girls, the mantra is "Open, DON'T BITE!" We found a dental practice that welcomes people with special needs. They even use PECS pictures. Our kids need dental care, perhaps more than NT girls—a cavity for us means a hospital visit and general anesthesia. Avoiding cavities is a must. Between my three daughters, we have had one cavity. I attribute this to a diet that includes only water to drink, few chewy/gummy snacks, and diligent brushing twice per day. We use Tom's fluoride-free toothpaste, and I allowed a

BPA-free sealant at their early visits, weighing the risks of cavities and hospital visits with the sealant.

~

When looking for a dentist for your ASD child, search for those who specialize in ASD kids. If you do not have one of these specialists nearby focus on pediatric dentists as they will be more likely to have been exposed to special-needs kids and be better equipped to handle them. Some might even have specific days of the week when they only schedule children with special needs. Also don't neglect the all important parent network—ask the parents of your child's classmates for references.

~

If your child has an object that he particularly loves (a music player or clock, for example), bring one with you to the dental visit so that the dentist can incorporate that into the appointment.

—Ruby Gelman, DMD

~

I have found that short, more-frequent visits prove to be very successful in the dental office. I will recommend seeing autistic kids every two to four months, and at each visit, we do the same things we did at the visit before, while incorporating something new each time. Kids will remember things better from one visit to the next.

—Ruby Gelman, DMD

~

On June 12, 2008, the FDA admitted on its website that silver fillings in our teeth are toxic and harmful to our health, and that they "might have neuro-toxic effects on the nervous systems of developing children and fetuses." Avoid them. Likewise, research fluoride before allowing fluoride treatments or using fluoride toothpaste.

~

Prevention is always the best medicine for colds and flu. Practice good hand washing and eating, drinking, and sleeping well; plus, a little knowledge about treatment options will go a long way.

Anesthesia and Your Child

Your child might require anesthesia for dental or surgical procedures. Many people with autism have unusual responses to anesthesia. Ask to meet the anesthesiologist several days before the procedure. Print out and bring the advice of Dr. Louise Kirz, an anesthesiologist with two children on the spectrum (http:// legacy.autism.com/ families/life/kirz.htm).

~

The following tips are adapted from the article "Anesthesia and the Autistic Child" by Sym C. Rankin, RN, CRNA, MS, *The Autism File*, Issue 33, 2009.

Anesthesia is unavoidable for children who need to undergo surgical procedures. The goal in such cases is to minimize the risk. To do that, the anesthesia provider must be made aware of the unique problems your child has.

- Your child may have gastrointestinal dysfunction, immune system dysregulation, inflammation, mitochondrial dysfunction, heavy metal poisoning, oxidative stress, and chronic inflammation.
- Most importantly, your child probably has impaired detoxification systems and may not be able to metabolize drugs efficiently.

~

When your child is scheduled to undergo a procedure, consider discussing the following issues during the preoperative conference:

- Ask not to use nitrous oxide. Most of our kids have a documented B12 deficiency.
- Discuss specific medical and metabolic problems concerning your child. Tell your provider of any genetic, methylation, detoxification, and mitochondrial issues.
- Consider placement of an IV without sedation. Many of our children undergo multiple blood draws and intravenous treatments. If your child can tolerate an IV placement, let your anesthesiologist know that because the provider usually will not expect children to tolerate this procedure.
- Inform the anesthesia provider of all medications, supplements, and IgE allergies.

- Make sure the provider understands that your child has difficulty detoxifying drugs.
- Ask the provider to keep the anesthetic as simple as possible.
- Discuss any other drugs that might be given in conjunction with the anesthetics (e.g., acetaminophen, steroids, and antiemetics).

Preventing Autism

The following tips was adapted from the article "Avoiding Autism" by Anju Usman, MD, and Beth C. Hynes, JD, MBA, *The Autism File*, Issue 31, 2009.

Due to the symbiotic relationship between a mother and her developing fetus, care must be taken by the mom before, during, and after pregnancy (if nursing) to both avoid exposure to harmful elements and to promote optimal maternal detoxification processes so that the host body remains as clean an environment as possible, within which vigorous infant development can unfold. Considering this, basic principles to guide you in decision-making surrounding pregnancy are as follows:

- You are what you eat (and drink); therefore, make healthy choices in what you consume.
- Skin is the largest organ in the body, so be very careful about what you rub into yours and your baby's.
- Think beyond "green." What is "green" for the environment is not always what is healthiest for the

body,but what is healthiest for the body is always "green."

Pre-Pregnancy

While planning a pregnancy, we recommend that you clean up any toxicity in your body and begin to follow a more-organic, healthy lifestyle. Remember, the less toxic you are, the better it is for you and your future baby. Undertake a sequential detoxification program that targets the liver and colon; this type of program can take six months or more and should not be done while pregnant.

~

In a careful manner, with an experienced dentist, remove amalgams from your teeth, which also can take six months or more.

~

Take the time now to find organic, nontoxic makeup, hair, and body products that you like and start integrating them into your daily life.

~

Ask your doctor to run some tests to determine any additional specific supplementation you may need to optimize levels within your body.

~

Remove all harmful chemical cleaning agents from your cleaning routine at home and at the office, and instead use cleaning products labeled "Level 1" by the EPA. Do not forget to include products for dishwashing and clothing detergent in your cleanup, and avoid toxic dry cleaning as much as possible.

~

Improve your nutrition with a targeted vitamin supplementation program to include omega-3 essential fatty acids, sublingual methyl B-12, folinic acid, vitamin D3, zinc, and antioxidants.

~

Eat organic, hormone-free food and avoid consuming fish or foods with MSG or food dyes.

~

Drink organic green tea, filtered water, and antioxidant-rich organic juices while avoiding soda, carbonated beverages, and alcohol.

~

Use Stevia, raw organic honey, and xylitol as sweeteners. Avoid any artificial sweeteners.

~

Go for walks and get some sunshine daily.

~

Cosmetics: use aluminum-free natural deodorant, natural hennas to color hair, and avoid moisturizers or makeup with chemicals or parabens in them. Also avoid chemical dyes, perms, or other such hair treatments.

~

Use only chemical-free cleaning products in your home, and avoid using pesticides or chemicals to treat your lawn.

During Pregnancy

Avoid medications to the extent possible, including acetaminophen, because it hinders normal detoxification. Avoid the flu vaccine, which contains mercury, a neurotoxin that can affect the baby's brain development. See http://www.safeminds.org/protect-yourself-2/flu-facts/.

~

Add zinc, calcium, essential fatty acids, and prenatal vitamins to your daily supplement intake.

~

Discontinue use of nail polish and any makeup (including lipstick) products that contain parabens and other toxins.

~

Use fluoride-free toothpaste, as fluoride interferes with iodine metabolism.

~

Do yoga and engage in stress management techniques, such as massage and listening to soothing music. Do not, however, start a rigorous exercise program, sit in a sauna, or get dental work (not even cleanings).

~

Get the mercury-free RhoGAM if you need this intervention. Eat fermented foods, cook with organic coconut oil, use organic raw apple cider as salad dressing, and consume healthy fats and cold pressed oil. Avoid fast food or seafood (especially tuna), and food packaged in plastic or styrofoam. Do not use a microwave.

~

Use a corded headset while talking on a cell phone. Don't work with a laptop computer on your lap.

Infancy

If you have amalgams and plan to nurse, you should send a sample of your breast milk to a specialty lab for heavy-metal testing.

~

If you plan to use formula, use those containing DHA (docosahexanenoic acid), an essential fatty acid critical to the healthy development of the central nervous system.

~

When introducing food, use organic baby food. Avoid the introduction of soy, gluten, or dairy until after the baby turns two years of age. After one year, supplement your baby's food with a quarter of a teaspoon of mercury-free cod liver oil.

~

For fevers over 101°F, treat with a tepid bath or dye-free ibuprofen. Fevers, while nerve-wracking for new parents, are the response of a healthy immune system reacting to kill off an invading virus through heat.

~

Antibiotics should be used sparingly and only for confirmed bacterial infections (they do not alleviate viral infections). Remember, antibiotic use disrupts the normal gut flora and promotes the overgrowth of yeast and resistant organisms that, in turn, harms the optimal functioning of the immune system. Bear in mind that most ear infections are viral and are thus not treatable with antibiotics. Use homeopathic ear drops to help ease the symptoms associated with ear infections and colds.

~

Use an organic baby mattress, bedding, pillows, and hypoallergenic encasements. Avoid pajamas soaked in flame-retardant chemicals.

~

Feed your baby using glass bottles, avoiding plastic bottles and cups; also avoid microwaving formula or breast milk.

~

Before vaccinating your child, take the following precautions:

- Read up on your rights to refuse vaccination according to your state's exemption laws. Visit www.nvic.org for a state by state map. As the parent, you have the right to make informed choices for your baby. That includes vaccination choice. If your pediatrician refuses, find another doctor. Ask other Moms who are altering the vaccine schedule (or choosing no vaccines at all) which docs are amenable to parental choice.

- If your child has a fever, constipation, diarrhea, or other illness, hold off on the vaccination.

- If your child is on antibiotics, hold off on the vaccination.

- If your child has an immune system disorder, allergies, or if they had a reaction to an earlier vaccine, hold off on the vaccine and seek another opinion.

- Know what the possible reactions are to each vaccine given.

- Immediately report side effects to your doctor.

- Remember to ask for single-dose mercury-free vaccines.

- Check titers before boosters, as they may not be necessary.

~

Vaccination is a "third rail" topic. I can't imagine the plight of a newly pregnant woman as she tries to sort fact from fear-inducing fiction. I suggest the following books for additional information to help you make healthcare choices for your daughter, some vaccines or no vaccines:

- *The Vaccine Book: Making the Right Decisions for Your Child* by Dr. Bob Sears
- *Vaccines 2.0: The Careful Parents' Guide to Making Safe Vaccination Choices* by Mark Blaxill and Dan Olmsted.

My girls are in the Gardasil age group. They have never, and will never receive this three-shot series. Gardasil is the Merck vaccine for HPV, the genital warts virus. GlaxoSmithKline has a version called Cevarix. My friend and colleague Mark Blaxill wrote a series called, "Gardasil, A License to Kill," that walks the reader through the collaboration between the government and Merck to bring this vaccine to market. I tell you this not to scare you—the pro-vaccine industry does a fine job of screaming "BOO!" at every turn. Every parent deserves information to make personal choices.

CHAPTER 4

Supporting the Family Unit

"How do you do it, Kim?" How do YOU do it, reader? How do any of us weather the daily ups and downs, grind, tears, and frustrations of raising a daughter with autism? Has anyone ever said to you, "Oh, you must be a SAINT!" Your eyes roll back into your head, right? I've heard that so many times that I wrote a memoir titled, *All I Can Handle: I'm No Mother Teresa*. None of us are. Nor do we have to be good parents, caretakers, therapists, or teachers.

Parents of typical kids get the pleasure and reward of watching their kids gain skills in a natural way as they grow into adulthood. Sweet sixteens and driver's licenses and SATs and weddings and grandbabies. No. No. No. No. Aaand no. Not here.

My girls make progress, but it sure isn't typical. And I admit that I feel a deep sadness and longing for the typical milestones of parenting. It gets harder, not easier once the kids become young adults. I expect that the girls' father and I will plunge into abject terror as we become elderly. So we have that to look forward to, right? Many readers will have typical kids in addition to a girl with autism. It can't be easy to juggle the two worlds.

So, what to do to combat this never-ending exhaustion and anxiety that could take Godzilla down, especially over time? I implore parents to find some sort of personal outlet. Something just for you. Preferably something whereby you can see and track improvement. You've seen the hokey sign: "If Mama ain't happy, ain't nobody happy." It's kind of true. We need to stay reasonably healthy and sane, and we deserve something just for ourselves.

Pick something—golf, knitting, tennis, yoga, ceramics, sword swallowing, karate. I picked karate. In 2010, I was sitting at the very same cramped desk in my eating area when two masked men broke into my garage and came into my house not twenty feet from where I am writing now. I heard the breaking glass and realized that "a crime was in progress" and snuck out the front door as they were opening the door from the garage. The police came and caught one robber who went to prison for a couple of years.

I felt so exposed and vulnerable that I knew I had to make some changes. I found a local karate school and started kickboxing. A few months later, I put on a gi and started training in Shito Ryu Karate-do. Today I'm a brown belt and I hope to earn my black belt within two years. Karate gives me fitness, strength, and flexibility, as well as self-defense skills for myself and my girls. And the belt system gives me tangible feedback for my progress. I like it. I need it.

Try to find something just for you. It's not selfish. It's self-preservation.

Self-Care

Self-care is imperative for parents so that they are available to their child to help them develop the key components for social, emotional, and intellectual development, including the ability to focus and attend, engage, interact, and use ideas creatively and logically.

—Lauren Tobing-Puente, PhD, "Parent Support,"
Cutting-Edge Therapies for Autism

~

Parents living with autism experience greater stress than other parents. Autism is 24/7, and if you don't give yourself a break, no one else will. You can't really help your daughter who has autism unless you take care of yourself first. Like they tell you on the airlines, you need to put on your own oxygen mask before you can help your child. Make sure you take breaks, even if it is just fifteen minutes to read the paper or catch a quick nap. Organize a weekly or monthly date with your partner or spouse, or a night out with the girls or guys. You deserve it. Besides, if you don't keep up with your social skills, how will you teach your daughter any?

—Chantal Sicile-Kira, www.chantalsicile-kira.com

~

It's essential that you take care of yourself and your needs, including giving yourself the time and space to grieve. You have lost the child you imagined you would have, and it's perfectly okay to mourn that loss. Mourn, but also discover the incredible new child you've been given. Eventually, those memories of that other child will fade and be replaced with the magnificent memories you will undoubtedly make.

~

Run! No, not away from your troubles but as a way to deal with them. You need exercise to keep fit for battle, and nothing is easier, cheaper, or more fun than running. Running is also a bona fide stress reliever and provides an opportunity for your mind to organize its thoughts. Join a local running club or organization. Here in New York City, we are blessed with the New York Road Runners, but there are many similar organizations around the country and if one is not near, start an affiliate!

Marriage Tips

A positive attitude will help. Today, marriages fall apart for a variety of reasons; and with an autistic child, however good and kind you might be in dealing with your child, it is exhausting, and the result is that it will take its toll on your marriage. So you need to adopt a positive frame of mind, and come up with solutions that will help both you and your spouse to spend quality time together.

—Abhishek Agarwal, www.health–whiz.com/555/index.htm

~

You will need to rediscover yourselves, and dwell on how you first met, what attracted you to each other, and try to remember each other's good points. Also, the autistic child needs to interact with other people as well, like a qualified nanny or a grandparent, even an uncle or aunt. This will definitely help the child to have a few other people in his life and be able to give you the break that you need, allowing you to spend more time with each other.

—Abhishek Agarwal, www.health-whiz.com/555/index.htm

~

Work together to save your marriage. Try to see what works best for your autistic child, and work together instead of blaming each other. Although it can be frustrating at times, you could agree to work on solutions that could help, and in the long run, it will be beneficial to both parents and child. Never try to medicate the child without first consulting a specialist. Prioritize your needs by keeping a certain time each week for time together as a family, especially if one parent spends most of their time with the child.

—Abhishek Agarwal, www.health-whiz.com/555/index.htm

~

Another important factor is the need to interact with other parents of autistic children; this way, you will be able to see how they deal with situations and exchange ideas which will help everyone. Always remember that you do not have to struggle alone; there is always help in the form of family, counselors, and fellow parents. By keeping the right perspective and a positive attitude, you can give your child the care and love he needs, as well as retain the spark in your marriage.

—Abhishek Agarwal, www.health-whiz.com/555/index.htm

~

When having a party, ask family members to help out. Organize a rotating team of adults, where each individual spends a half hour with the child. This allows parents and siblings to enjoy themselves, and the child doesn't have to be exposed to the chaos of the party.

Counseling and Support Groups

Parents should be as much the focus in treatment as the children themselves, as their well-being is critical to their ability to be a part of their children's therapy. The optimal functioning of the parents is essential if the treatment strategies are to be successfully implemented.

—Lauren Tobing-Puente, PhD, "Parent Support," *Cutting-Edge Therapies for Autism*

~

A support system is crucial—and not just a family-and-friends system, but a group of people familiar with autism who might be able to help you out with the intricacies of the condition.

~

No one can do autism alone. Find friends—they are necessary for survival.

—Judith Chinitz, MS, MS, CNC, author of *We Band of Mothers*

Siblings

Look for support groups that support not only parents, but also siblings. You should also consider counseling. Talk with your pediatrician and your health-care professional to establish whether counseling is necessary; if the autistic child receives most of a parent's attention, her siblings might feel left out.

—www.adviceaboutautism.com/treating-autism-at-home.html

~

Set aside time to spend with your typical child(ren). They should have their "alone" time with each parent where each can focus on their needs and interests.

~

Siblings should have their own safe place, out of the way when you need to settle down or focus on your child with autism who may be melting down. After things calm down, return to your typical child and help him or her understand what occurred.

Friends and Family

Sometimes we feel uncomfortable when a good friend or relative has a child with autism, because we don't know how to react or what to say. Here are some tips from *41 Things to Know about Autism* by Chantal Sicile-Kira (www.chantalsicile-kira.com):

- If you were good friends before the diagnosis and were in contact often, don't change. Your friend may not have the free time they had before to see you, but you can stay connected by phone or e-mail. Keep those lines of communication open.

- Stay connected by continuing to invite them over. If they can come, they'll come; if they can't, they won't. It can be hard for them to get out of the house, but don't give up, and keep the invitations coming.

- Find out a little bit about autism. Go to reputable websites and get some basic information.

- Learn more than you advise. It can be tempting to tell them everything you hear about autism in the news, but your friend has probably heard it all. Instead, offer an ear and some practical help.

- Is there some way you can help by offering them some precious time? They may not need advice, but they could sure use a break. Could you watch the child with autism for a few hours? Or maybe take the siblings out? How about dropping off a home-cooked meal one night?

- Don't ignore the child with autism because you don't know how to connect with her. Follow her lead and show interest in what she is doing. Show her something she might like. You can ask the parents for tips on how to interact withher; they will surely appreciate the overtures.

~

Convey helpful hints to others who will be interacting with your child. For example, suggest that they:

- Speak slowly and use simple language
- Use concrete terms
- Repeat simple questions
- Allow time for responses
- Give lots of praise
- Do not attempt to physically block self-stimulating behavior
- Remember that each individual with autism is unique and may act differently than others

~

The child or teen with autism may look like they are not paying attention, but they are taking in everything that is going on around them. They are listening to you even if they are not looking at you. Not being able to talk does not mean they don't understand you, or that they have nothing to communicate. Treat each child as if they understand what is being said in their presence. Give them the benefit of the doubt.

—Chantal Sicile-Kira, www.chantalsicile-kira.com

Home Help

As with most services, I have found the best sitters and helpers from other parents. You can also ask around at your child's school, camp, or play group. Many times some of the folks who work with the kids during the day are available to work at your home, either performing therapy or just supervising while you are out for a night of respite.

~

Check out your local colleges, which will usually post your sitter requests with the appropriate department, possibly in the special-needs education department.

~

Once you hire someone, you want to keep them if they are good. Here are some tips on supervising people to work in your home with your daughter:

- Make sure the responsibilities are clear, including the times you are expecting them, and that they are responsible for communicating any changes to you as soon as possible.
- Have a calendar—in the kitchen or online—easily available where people can see special appointments or changes in scheduling.
- If you expect some degree of flexibility on their part, be prepared to be flexible for them.
- Make sure you have everything they need to do their work, and that everything has a specific place so things are easily found.
- Remember that they are there to help your child and not to be your counselor. Don't overburden them with all the problems you are having with, say, the school district.
- Remember to keep boundaries—keep your rapport with them respectful and professional.
- Have high expectations of their job performance, but make sure you have what they need to get the job done.

—Chantal Sicile-Kira, www.chantalsicile-kira.com

CHOCOLATE CHIP COOKIES

This is my go-to recipe for the All-American comfort treat, the chocolate chip cookie. It's from the *Rosie's Bakery All-Butter, Fresh Cream, Sugar Packed, No-Holds Barred Baking Book* by Judy Rosenberg of Boston's Rosie's Bakery. ©1991 Workman Publishing.

Two simple ingredient swaps create an equally yummy GF/CF version.

2 cups plus 1 tablespoon all purpose flour (or Pamela's Artisan GF flour blend)

1 teaspoon baking soda

¾ teaspoon salt

1 cup (2 sticks) butter (or Spectrum butter flavored shortening)

1 cup light brown sugar

½ cup plus 2 tablespoons granulated sugar

1 teaspoon vanilla extract (GF if needed)

2 eggs, room temp

1½ cup chocolate chips (Enjoy Life brand is dairy free.)

Preheat oven to 375°F. Sift flour, baking soda, and salt into small bowl, set aside. (I am too lazy to sift, FYI.) In mixing bowl, cream the softened butter or shortening with the brown and white sugar and then add the eggs. Scrape the bowl a few times. Add the dry ingredients and mix on low until blended. Add the chips. Use a small ice cream scoop or melon ball scoop to place onto baking sheet. Bake 11 to 12 minutes. Cool on rack. Hide in freezer!

CHAPTER 5
Daily Life

Daily Life covers a lot of ground. We have to think about every facet of our girls' lives. Parents of typical kids find that once a skill is taught or comes naturally (yeah, that happens I hear . . . never seen it), they can check that skill off the "to teach" list and move onto the next set of skills. Are you laughing out loud? We have to teach, reteach, unteach, teach, and reteach daily living skills throughout our girls' lives. Take the deep breath and allow yourself to make mistakes; you have your daughter's full lifetime to help her.

Teaching Basic Skills

Begin teaching independence and daily living skills early on. It might take your child some time to perfect them. It's better to start earlier than later. Try things like having them set the table for dinner or preparing their own lunch.

—Megan Miller, Head Teacher

~

Get your child involved. Even if your child cannot complete the entire task, break down daily routines to give them a role. For example, give your child a shoelace to pull when untying laces, fasten the zipper and then allow your child to finish the task by pulling the zipper up, etc. add more steps as your child's skills develop to further increase his/her independence.

—Jenn Gross, OTR/L

Improving Communication Skills

Remember that behavior is communication. If a nonverbal child has no communication system, they will learn to communicate inappropriate behaviors. Often educators and parents are hesitant to use alternative systems of communications (i.e., PECS, typing, sign language) because they are afraid it will hinder speech developing, or that it is like giving up on their child or student. However, research has proven just the opposite: these alternative communication methods enhance the child's ability to speak.

—Chantal Sicile-Kira, www.chantalsicile-kira.com

~

Show your child what you mean. Children who have difficulty comprehending language often watch what others are doing very carefully—at least, when they are interested. If you are going to show your child something, you can say "Watch!" You should be saying "Just watch! I will show you" so often that your child tunes right in when you say this, and watches what you do next. Teach your child to watch when told to watch by doing very interesting things after you say it.

—Tahirih Bushey MA-CCC, Autism Games,
http://sites.google.com/site/autismgames/home/parent-tips

~

When pursuing augmentative and alternative communication (AAC) solutions for a nonverbal child, it's important to remember that such solutions rarely work in isolation. Though universally associated with electronic speech-generating technology, AAC includes self-expressive strategies that we all use naturally, such as writing, gestures, and eye contact. Simple AAC tools—from picture symbol cards to digital photographs imported to a speech-generating device or organized in a scrapbook—can help keep communication predictable and meaningful for your child. Successful communication often happens when use of multiple modalities (including your child's verbal approximations) coincides with realistic expectations from typically speaking communication partners.

—Patti Murphy, Writer, DynaVox Mayer-Johnson

~

Some autistic individuals do not know that speech is used for communication. Language learning can be facilitated if language exercises promote communication. If the child asks for a cup, then give him a cup. If the child asks for a plate, when he wants a cup, give him a plate. The individual needs to learn that when he says words, concrete things happen. It is easier for an individual with autism to learn that their words are wrong if the incorrect word resulted in the incorrect object.

—Temple Grandin, PhD, author of
Thinking in Pictures and *The Way I See It*,
www.autism.com/ind_teaching_tips.asp

~

Children who have difficulty understanding speech have a hard time differentiating between hard consonant sounds such as "D" in dog and "L" in log. My speech teacher helped me to learn to hear these sounds by stretching out and enunciating hard consonant sounds. Even though the child might have passed a pure-tone hearing test, he might still have difficulty hearing hard consonants. Children who talk in vowel sounds are not hearing consonants.

—Temple Grandin, PhD, author of
Thinking in Pictures and *The Way I See It*,
www.autism.com/ind_teaching_tips.asp

~

Avoid long strings of verbal instructions. People with autism have problems with remembering the sequence. If the child can read, write the instructions down on a piece of paper. I am unable to remember sequences. If I ask for directions at a gas station, I can only remember three steps. Directions with more than three steps have to be written down. I also have difficulty remembering phone numbers because I cannot make a picture in my mind.

> —Temple Grandin, PhD, author of
> *Thinking in Pictures* and *The Way I See It*,
> www.autism.com/ind_teaching_tips.asp

~

Some children and adults can sing better than they can speak. They might respond better if words and sentences are sung to them. Some children with extreme sound sensitivity will respond better if the teacher talks to them in a low whisper.

> —Temple Grandin, PhD, author of
> *Thinking in Pictures* and *The Way I See It*,
> www.autism.com/ind_teaching_tips.asp

Improving Social Skills

Children with autism do not naturally know how to ask for help, and this is a social skill that needs to be taught. For example, at recess, if a little child's shoelace becomes undone, the child will naturally go to ask the teacher for help in tying it up again. Not so the child with autism. You can teach this with children when they are requesting something they are having difficulty opening or reaching by pairing it with the spoken word or icon. Then, teaching them to come looking for you when they need help is the next step.

> —Chantal Sicile-Kira, www.chantalsicile-kira.com

~

When your daughter is little, you can arrange playdates for her. As she gets older, you will have to teach her how to initiate contact with others, such as how to call and arrange to meet someone, how to send a text message, or leave a voice-mail message. Encourage her to find clubs at school to join, like chess, animal- related clubs, or drama.

~

Many girls with autism are enjoying the use of Facebook to communicate or learn about other people, even if they need help to do so. Those who have little verbal skills find this a good way to connect with others.

~

Teach girls that the correct distance that a person should be standing from another is an arm's length away. It is rude for the girl to get closer than that unless it is a family member. Conversely, unless is someone is very well-known to them, they should not get closer than an arm's length to the girl. Parents can amend this rule to add exceptions as the girl gets older.

~

Teenage girls and adult women need to learn and practice safety rules for social situations, such as where and when to make dates or appointments with people they do not know well. They need to learn the rule that they should meet in the daytime in places where there are bound to be people around (i.e., Starbucks, the campus library or coffee shop) and never at night and in private places.

~

What has been helpful for teenage girls and women with autism is to have a trustworthy female they know well with whom they can "practice" social situations. They make the rule that they will run situations by this person to get feedback on appropriateness to avoid possibly bad situations.

~

To prevent teenage girls from giving the wrong "signal," teach them that staring at certain parts of another's anatomy is rude and inappropriate. The rule should be that a person should never stare at the private parts of another person's body, the area normally covered by a bathing suit (male or female).

~

An ASD teen girl may not be able to "read" the cues from another person as to whether the interest is reciprocal. The teen needs to have explicit instruction about indications that someone likes them, as opposed to being interested romantically.

~

At school, find the girls who are naturally the "mother hens," as they can take your daughter under their wings and help her to learn the rules of social behavior at school. In this way, your daughter will become more adept in social situations at school.

~

The "hidden curriculum"—the unstated rules in social situations—is something that needs to be taught to girls with autism, as they don't pick it up by osmosis like the other girls. As teens, it can become even more challenging. A good resource to help teach them what they need to know is *The Hidden Curriculum: Practical Solutions for Understanding Unstated Rules in Social Solutions* by Brenda Smith-Myles, et al.

~

Talking to the teen girl can help demystify the change in their classmates' behavior from mainly same-sex interaction, to mixed interaction, with flirting, touching, showing off for the benefit of potential boyfriends. This helps them to make sense of what is going on around them, as they don't pick that up by osmosis. It will help them to understand that behaviors such as teasing, playful punching, etc., may be an indication of flirting rather than an offense that needs to be reported to the teacher.

~

Teach the girl the difference between private and public conversations. Private conversations (i.e., talking about your period) are for private places (home) with close family (your sister and mom). Public conversations (shopping, homework, hairstyles) are okay in public places (school cafeteria) with public people (your classmates).

Improving Reading Skills

The following tips are adapted from "11 Tips to Encourage Reading in Children with Autism" by Alice Woolley, www. insidethebubble.co.uk.

~

Read daily and follow up. Try to get into the habit of some daily reading, because you want your child to remember what he learned the previous day, and to build on it.

~

Even a little daily reading does the trick. Don't put it all off until the weekend, and then attempt a marathon literacy session. It is far easier to concentrate for a short space of time, depending on the age of your child and his normal attention span. You might need to start at just five minutes at a time, increasing as your child gets older to around forty-five minutes; beyond that time, you will get less and less return for your efforts.

~

Use "cvc" (consonant-vowel-consonant) words first. Many books for children, even early board books and first readers, will not be designed with your child's vocabulary in mind. Some of them even include words that children at the earliest reading levels will not have a hope of being able to pronounce, such as "xylophone" or "through." Three-letter cvc words are among the easiest to pronounce. Ensure that any material you give your child early on has plenty of these.

~

Rhyme and repetition: *The Cat in the Hat* by Dr. Seuss is a good book for beginners due to its repetition of "cvc" rhyming words. Repeated words are obviously easier to remember.

~

Start with words that are pronounced as they are spelled. Even some short words aren't pronounced phonetically; for example, words such as what, was, two, girl, one, and are. Avoid dealing with these words until your child is fairly confident with words that are pronounced the way they are written. When she is successfully reading words such as cat, bin, or get, gradually introduce words with more difficult pronunciations.

~

Persevere. Although it's not uncommon for children with autism to experience reading difficulties, it's also not unknown for an apparently hopeless situation to turn around as soon as they reach the right stage of development. Sometimes, things just click into place.

~

Don't let your child guess. Sometimes your child will take clues about what she is reading from the surrounding pictures.

Also, if she is overly familiar with a story, she might simply remember how it goes without having to read. In order to assess her true reading level, you will sometimes need to use text, and to vary the stories frequently. Again, this is where a chalkboard or text-only flashcards will come in handy.

—

Several parents have informed me that using the closed captions on the television helped their child to learn to read. The child was able to read the captions and match the printed words with spoken speech. Recording a favorite program with captions on a tape would be helpful because the tape can be played over and over again and stopped.

—Temple Grandin, PhD, author of *Thinking in Pictures* and
The Way I See It,
ww.autism.com/ind_teaching_tips.asp

Improving Academic Skills

Many autistic children get fixated on one subject, such as trains or maps. The best way to deal with fixations is to use them to motivate schoolwork. If the child likes trains, then use trains to teach reading and math. Read a book about a train and do math problems with trains. For example, calculate how long it takes for a train to go between new York and Washington.

—Temple Grandin, PhD, author of
Thinking in Pictures and *The Way I See It*,
www.autism.com/ind_teaching_tips.asp

~

Let children look for an object in warmed sand or discriminate between several objects in sand by touching. Exercise explorative touching, without eye contact, with two-dimensional shapes as a pre-exercise for visual exploration of letters and other forms.

—Bob Woodward and Dr. Marga Hogenboom,
Autism: A Holistic Approach

~

Use concrete visual methods to teach number concepts. My parents gave me a math toy that helped me to learn numbers. It consisted of a set of blocks that had a different length and a different color for the numbers one through ten. With this I learned how to add and subtract. To learn fractions my teacher had a wooden apple that was cut up into four pieces and a wooden pear that was cut in half. From this I learned the concept of quarters and halves.

—Temple Grandin, PhD, author of
Thinking in Pictures and *The Way I See It*,
www.autism.com/ind_teaching_tips.asp

~

Some individuals with autism will respond better and have improved eye contact and speech if the teacher interacts with them while they are swinging on a swing or rolled up in a mat. Sensory input from swinging or pressure from the mat sometimes helps to improve speech. Swinging should always be done as a fun game. It must never be forced.

—Temple Grandin, PhD, author of
Thinking in Pictures and *The Way I See It*,
www.autism.com/ind_teaching_tips.asp

Homework Tips

The following tips are provided by Cathy Purple Cherry, AIA, LEED AP.

~

Our nineteen-year-old autistic son is on a certificate track, not a diploma track, at his school. Our focus now for his education is life skills and independence. He is at a 4th grade math level and 7th grade English level. My tips come from raising this autistic child.

~

Once our son got into middle school, I needed to figure out what I felt was important for his education and future. Don't look just to the day or year. As a parent of an autistic child, look far forward into their adulthood. This significantly impacts the educational decisions you make and the way you advocate during his or her school years.

~

Strong communication with your ASD child's teachers and special educational coordinator is pivotal. You should use email and document, document, document. Keep this correspondence as well as it may be needed for reference in future IEP meetings. My son was an A student but would only answer one of ten questions on a sheet of paper. For me, it was important to have documentation from the teacher that he got his A's for effort only because I felt his grades misrepresented his processing abilities to the Board of Education.

~

Determine from your child's teachers how much time they want spent on homework. I got to the place where each teacher wrote at the top of their assignments the amount of time to be spent on the piece. I then sat my son down, set a timer, and when it went off, I stopped his efforts. It did not matter if he had only processed one question. Homework in an autistic child's world, in my opinion, is not nearly as important as him doing things he likes to do or doing things that help prepare him for independence. And more significantly, the sanity of the whole family is far more important than completing struggling homework.

~

Assess your child's academic gifts and work with these. Do not angst over making your child perform academically in an area of education that he or she is not good at. Know that time is the best teacher for these kids and that all things with them take more time. End of story. Do NOT do your child's homework believing you are helping him or her. This can give a false impression to his educational team and come back to haunt you in his IEP meetings.

~

Tips for Helping an ADHD with Homework (also applies to children with ASDs), by Laura Wilson, http:// adhdchildren.suite101.com/article.cfm/tips-for-helping-an-adhd-child-with-homework.

- For a child to get her homework done, she will need an environment conducive to studying. First, make sure the student has all materials at hand. A child with ADHD who has to wander off to find an eraser will have a difficult time settling down to concentrate again. Second, figure out what noise level is helpful for the student. Some children work best in absolute silence. Others need some white noise like the whir of a fan in the background. Even some types of music can help a child's productivity. Parents will need to experiment with different options, and then stick with what works best.

- Now that the routine and environment are set, parents can add in some other variables to see if they help the child.

- Allow a child to stand if sitting makes her jittery. The ability to move around a bit might help her concentrate. Use a square of tape on the floor to make a box for her feet if she wanders too much.

- Provide textures to aid in productivity. Attach some adhesive Velcro strips (soft side) to the desk for the child to rub her hand on, or make some stress balls of

balloons filled with flour, rice, or sugar for the child to
play with while she's thinking.

- Certain scents aid in concentration. Experiment with
basil, pine, peppermint, or citrus scents to see if any of
these help.

- Keep the mouth busy. For some children, chewing
gum or snacking on something crunchy (like apples or
crackers) can help productivity.

- Check on the child often, before she goes too far down
the wrong road. It's frustrating to have to do a whole
assignment over, but if a parent can see a problem
before it goes on too long, it won't be such a big deal.

- Give rewards. As with many parenting challenges,
rewarding exceptional effort or work will motivate the
child to continue to do his best.

- A student with Attention Deficit Disorder can
be successful and productive during homework
time. Parents who help their child create a positive
environment and routine will see great results when
used in cooperation with helpful strategies.

- Allow breaks after a predetermined amount of time. For
example, set a timer for fifteen minutes for a younger
child, and allow her a five-minute break to stretch, run
around, or play with a pet. Their work time will be
more productive in short segments.

~

In addition to establishing and maintaining a routine and
plan for communicating with a child's teacher, parents must
also reinforce routines at home. As autistic children and

adults often struggle with high issues of anxiety and worry, parents can help assuage feelings of angst by adhering to a daily program and regimen.

—Grace Chen, "5 Tips for Helping Your Autistic Child Excel in Public Schools," www.publicschoolreview.com/articles/88

Managing Your Child's Environment

Become an expert on your child. Figure out what triggers your kid's "bad" or disruptive behaviors and what elicits a positive response. What does your autistic child find stressful? Calming? Uncomfortable? Enjoyable? If you understand what affects your child, you'll be better at troubleshooting problems and preventing situations that cause difficulties.

—Reprinted with permission from helpguide.org. See www.helpguide.org/mental/autism_help.htm for additional resources and support.

Observe your child's behavior and mood following meals, environment changes (going outside during the summer), and exposure to different lighting, sounds, and sights. Become Sherlock Holmes to pinpoint situations that need adjusting.

~

If a child covers her ears playfully, ask if she likes loud sounds muffled through their hands, or quiet like a whisper. Then act out the question. Get her to indicate a preference and then thank her for helping you to do what makes her most comfortable. Now play with it! Tell her you like it sung and sing about your love for her. The idea is to desensitize and educate the sensory system while watching her cues and then teaching her to put words to her desires. Running from her actions as if you have hurt her with your exuberance will make it so.

—Lynette Louise, MS, Board certified in
Neurofeedback by BCIA, NTCB

~

Create a home safety zone. Carve out a private space in your home where your child can relax, feel secure, and be safe. This will involve organizing and setting boundaries in ways your child can understand. Visual cues can be helpful (colored tape marking areas that are off-limits, labeling items in the house with pictures). You might also need to safety-proof the house, particularly if your child is prone to tantrums or other self-injurious behaviors.

—Reprinted with permission from helpguide.org.
See www.helpguide.org/mental/autismhelp.htm
for additional resources and support.

~

Don't be afraid to discipline your child when necessary. It is important not to underestimate your child. Children with autism are capable of willful misbehavior. It can be a challenge to determine what is willful and what is not, but parents should not assume that all behaviors are unintentional. Much like a typical child, an autistic child can and should be told what she should or should not do.

Family Activities

Board games are fun for autistic children to play with parents and siblings. These children often gravitate toward games that involve logical and strategic thinking, such as memory games or puzzles. This type of activity allows the child to interact closely with family members.

—Angie Geisler, "Fun Activity Suggestions
for Parents of Children with Wutism,"
www.brighthub.com/education/special/
articles/57559.aspx#ixzz0l0Qc6jnt

~

When parents of children with autism regularly plan cooperative activities, they help to increase a child's confidence level and to foster the communication skills that are necessary for participation in activities with both autistic and neurotypical peers.

—Angie Geisler, "Fun Activity Suggestions
for Parents of Children with Autism,"
www.brighthub.com/education/special/
articles/57559.aspx#ixzz0l0Qc6jnt

~

Activities that focus on sensory exploration, particularly those that involve visual and tactile learning, can easily be organized in the home environment. Some sensory activities that children with autism respond well to include finger-painting, water-table play, matching color flashcards, building block structures, and using Play-Doh (not for children on a gluten-free diet). Parents can bond with their child and encourage two-way communication by actively participating in these activities rather than allowing the child to play alone.

—Angie Geisler, "Fun Activity Suggestions for Parents of Children with Autism," www.brighthub.com/education/special/ articles/57559.aspx#ixzz0l0Qc6jnt

Teaching Behavioral and "Social" Management

Make use of self-stimulating behaviors. While stimming is typically performed to gain a sensory escape or satisfy a physical need, if you join in during these periods you may gain a quick glance or other feedback and have the beginning of a communication to build on.

~

If your daughter is melting down or very upset, try to remain in a calm state and keep a steady, serene appearance. In many cases this can serve to calm her quicker than is typical.

~

If your child is hyperactive and out of control, don't be tempted to react by shouting to get her to stop; in an overcrowded or noisy location (playground, store), it is likely that the environment is over stimulating her to begin with, and shouting will only make things worse. Likewise, a sensation-craving kid might grab items off a store shelf or run around because the environment is so tempting and overwhelming to her regulatory ability. scolding will only add to the turmoil and lead to feelings of guilt (by both) later on. To calm the child and get her regulated, remove her from the location, and use a soothing activity . . . always remember to counterbalance a child's loss of control with calm words and gestures, and help the child reorganize and regain focus and attention.

—Stanley Greenspan, MD, *Overcoming ADHD*

~

Alternatively, the child might need you to be completely quiet.

~

Listen to your child's body language: is she running, jumping, crashing onto the floor or into the wall? Does she prefer sedentary activities? Talk to your child's occupational therapist about the movements and sensations that your child seeks. Ask for a sensory diet to give your child consistent input and help satisfy these "cravings."

—Jenn Gross, OTR/L

~

Put your child to work. Heavy work that includes resistive activities (such as pushing, pulling, and carrying) provides input that is organizing and calming. At home you can have your child help with everyday chores while providing this important information to the body. Examples: pushing in chairs after mealtimes, pushing shopping carts at the grocery store, carrying heavier food items (rice, cans, etc.) and helping to put them away, carrying boxes of games to clean up, pulling the laundry basket to the machine, etc.

—Jenn Gross, OTR/L

~

Allow your daughter a significant amount of time to process and think after asking them a question. Thinking is hard work, but crucial for their development.

—Megan Miller, Head Teacher

Computer and Device Time

Mia and Gianna could spend all day on their iPads. Much of that time would be pure stimming on YouTube videos of old Boobah episodes set to Swedish death metal music (amuse yourself, Google Boobah Dimmu Booghir and you'll know what my house sounds like) and the first eight seconds of any random Sesame Street video. Pause. Repeat. Pause. Repeat. Pause Repeat.

Bella uses her iPad for recreation at home and also to really communicate—but she does not have speech like her sisters. She uses an app called AVATalker, designed and marketed by my good friend Erik Nansteil. It's like the old PECS come to life in an easy to use, easy to build upon app. Check it out at the iTunes store.

~

Apps! Apps run on the iPhone, iTouch, and iPad, providing a range of choices for your child. There are literally hundreds of autism related apps—just search for autism in the app store. Some favorites include Proloquo2Go (a full-featured communication solution), Is That Gluten Free?, Learn to Talk, iPrompts, ABA Flash Cards, and iMean (which turns the entire screen into a large-button keyboard with text display).

~

For a blog that reviews autism-related apps, checkout autism epicenter: http://autismepicenter.net/blog/blog2.php/2010/06/01/autism-apps-that-will-help-you.

~

Choose when your child will use the computer intentionally, and, just like television, sparingly. The computer has the potential to be wonderfully educational and the potential to be terribly harmful to your child's social development.

—Tahirih Bushey MA-CCC, Autism Games, http://sites.google.com/site/autismgames/home/parent-tips

~

Use the computer as a social motivator rather than a break from social interaction. This means finding ways to interact with your child or help your child interact with others while using the computer, and insisting that the computer be used as a social tool.

—Tahirih Bushey MA-CCC, Autism Games,
http://sites.google.com/site/autismgames/home/parent-tips

~

Help your child use new knowledge or skills learned on the computer in other places and in social situations. For example, if your child is playing a Dora the Explorer computer game in which Dora is finding treasures, and Swiper tries to steal treasures periodically, then make up a game in which you find the same treasures with your child around the house. Don't skip this step; take the time to figure out how to do this generalization step for every new computer game you introduce to your child, if possible. It is the tendency of children with ASD to learn in a fragmented way, and not to make the connections between things learned in one setting to things learned in another setting. The computer can become like an alternative world, but the skills learned on the computer should become useful in the real world.

—Tahirih Bushey MA-CCC, Autism Games,
http://sites.google.com/site/autismgames/home/parent-tips

~

Beware that your resolve to limit computer use might weaken if you are not careful! Yes, the computer can teach your child new skills. And yes, your child might really enjoy time on the computer . . . but I have watched many parents struggle with a child who is addicted to the computer as though it were a drug. I have seen children who are willing to do violence to get more time on the computer. Uncontrolled use of the computer has a family-destroying potential similar to letting your child watch too many videos, or letting your child demand that you buy things whenever you shop, or letting your child's demands convince you to make him or her something different for dinner. There are certain predictable child demands that, if you give in to them, can make your family life very difficult and do more harm than good for your child. Uncontrolled computer use is one of these.

—Tahirih Bushey MA-CCC, Autism Games,
http://sites.google.com/site/autismgames/home/parent tips

~

The computer is a wonderful tool for us all, and many of us love our computers inordinately, but we all have to learn to use them moderately and wisely. it is easier to be proactive on this than make a change in family rules, but if need be, put the computer away for a while and start over with new rules a few months later.

—Tahirih Bushey MA-CCC, Autism Games,
http://sites.google.com/site/autismgames/home/parent-tips

~

Temple Grandin often says that letting your child or teen spend too much time on the computer without a purpose is not a good idea. You do want to encourage computer skills to develop, as they may lead to job or career possibilities. To do that, Temple suggests finding a mentor to come over once a week to teach different computer applications and develop skill areas that could be helpful for future employment.

—Chantal Sicile-Kira, www.chantalsicile-kira.com

Sleep Tips!

My Dad was born in 1922. He used to tell us about a product called "paragoric" used to make babies go to sleep. It was a tincture of opium. Nighty night! I am a holy terror when I don't get consistent sleep. The Geneva Convention prohibits abnormal sleep deprivation. The Geneva Convention never had a child with autism . . .

Sleep rules! Remember kids and parents perform better and will be happier with a good night's sleep. Do not allow medications or other treatments to limit this important function. Try melatonin if there are difficulties; it works for many kids on the spectrum and it is good for parents having trouble sleeping as well.

~

Chronic problems can occur in the absence of a consistent bedtime routine, which should include a specific bedtime and a clearly defined sleep location, both a bedroom and a bed.

—Ellen Notbohm and Veronica Zysk,
*1001 Great Ideas for Teaching and Raising Children
with Autism Spectrum Disorders*

~

Occasional sleep problems can result from many different sources and be difficult to analyze. Look at the possible side effects of any new medications, any change in diet, the need for a bowel movement, adjustments to schedule, or perhaps nap during the day. Once again a log of daily activities can help pinpoint the cause.

~

Blackout shades are a good option, and they have the added bonus of making bedrooms dark for deeper sleep during naps.

—Candi Summers, Autism & Parenting Examiner, examiner.com, http://exm.nr/9sfVh8

Sleeping Tips from Cathy Purple Cherry, AIA, LEED AP

Our son is now nineteen. He was adopted from Russia at three. He still rocks himself to sleep with a side to side motion. This motion is very soothing for him so we allow it to happen for a limited period of time. I have discovered that if I tell him to roll to his stomach, the rocking stops and he falls asleep faster. If you wonder why I limit the time, it is because he also goes to camp and school and has roommates. This motion and sound can be very frustrating to others. Thus, I teach them also to tell him to roll to his stomach after a few soothing minutes.

~

Recognize that even typically-developing children and mostly autistic children can't go from 60 mph to 0 mph in a short time limit. Thus, don't fool yourself to think you can just say, "Okay everyone. It's time for bed!" The time process related to preparing an autistic child for bed can be extensive due to the number of prompts required to take all the steps. Also, calm the house down well in advance of when you want to start the process by dimming or turning off lights and lowering noise levels from the TV or other children. For our family, I would say it took originally 2 hours for this process. Now, at his age of nineteen, I would say it takes a minimum of 30 minutes, but you must be firm in your voice tone to constantly move the child forward.

~

What works for each ASD child can be different. Try tucking the blankets tightly around the child or allow the child to sleep in his or her clothes. Watch carefully for what seems to be patterns and obsessions and work with or through these. Do not try to make the child comply with your definition of proper bedtime routines.

A body pillow or even a sleeping bag can fill in for you when it's time for your child to make the transition to sleeping on her own. If your daughter is resistant to sleeping without you, try placing such an item in the bed with her to take up the extra space.

~

Epsom salt baths. Give in the evening, and morning if time permits. Epsom salt promotes calming and acts as a mild chelator, pulling toxins from the body. It also promotes sleep.

~

Melatonin. Use at night, start with about 1 mg, increase the dose as weight increases. Use the slow-release formulation for night awakenings, standard formulation for trouble falling asleep. This supplement is very safe and easy to go on and off in comparison to sleep drugs. Side benefits include more mellow days (a good night's sleep does wonders) and antioxidant properties.

WORMS

Say what? Worms as part of a "Daily Life" chapter? In our household, pinworms have been a regular and unwanted house/gut guest. Many of our kids have compromised GI systems. Add in close contact with peers who share similar issues and you have a gut ripe for a pinworm infestation. Pinworms are a common parasite in typical toddlers. I can remember drinking a thick, blood-red medicine as a child for pinworms. They are tiny, ¼-inch-long thread-like worms. The females crawl down into the anus at night to lay their eggs. This crawling creates itching, irritability, and night waking. The worms hatch around the full moon, which also causes behaviors and night waking. Kids scratch, then suck their thumb or finger, and the life cycle continues.

If you suspect pinworms, at night use a flashlight to look at your child's rectum. If white wiggly threads appear, those are pinworms. Take a piece of clear cellotape and dab-dab-dab around the rectum and bring the tape to your pediatrician. He or she can look under a microscope to see if there are eggs on the tape. This is called "the tape test." You don't have to get fancy with fecal tests for pinworms, although fecal tests can be helpful determine if there are other parasites in the intestinal tract.

There are both allopathic and natural treatments for worms, which are notoriously hard to eradicate.

Chapter 6

Productive Approaches to Parenting

All the Time

Be consistent. Autistic children have a hard time adapting what they've learned in one setting (such as the therapist's office or school) to others, including the home. For example, your child might use sign language at school to communicate, but never think to do so at home. Creating consistency in your child's environment is the best way to reinforce learning. Find out what your child's therapists are doing and continue their techniques at home. It's also important to be consistent in the way you interact with your child and deal with challenging behaviors.

—Reprinted with permission from helpguide.org.
See www.helpguide.org/mental/autismhelp.htm
for additional resources and support.

~

Having autism does not mean your daughter cannot have a fulfilling life; do not allow the language of victimhood into your vocabulary. Use empowering words that teach her that she is without limits.

~

Work to give your child some structured chores she can work on each day. This will help increase the structure in her day and give her a feeling of accomplishment each day. We suggest placing play items in a home bin and helping with laundry.

~

Get control of your children while they are still little. What's bearable when they are three isn't so bearable when they have pubic hair.

—Judith Chinitz, MS, MS, CNC, author of *We Band of Mothers*

~

A clearly defined daily schedule for your daughter can work wonders to remove uncertainty and accompanying frustration, for you both!

~

Seek some good self time and solace. Go for a walk in the woods, run in the park, or read a book by a lake. You need to take care EXPAND of yourself and activities in nature have a tonic effect.

~

You must adjust the expectations you have for your child. Many children are expected to sit still through an entire dinner, but this is an unrealistic expectation for a child with autism. Begin with smaller, more attainable goals for your child. Make it a goal to sit at the table for five minutes, or use the correct utensil to eat with. Once these goals are reached, you can eventually move to sitting for an entire meal.

~

Flexibility is key, especially when it comes to timing. Knowing when to back off and when to return to a task or duty is more art than science. Keeping a flexible mindset and being persistent will help!

~

Early on, friendships between young girls are often very play-based. By the time they reach middle school, the friendships between girls shift to really be a lot about talking, chatting on the phone, texting. There's much more deep communicative talking, sharing thoughts and feelings. At this time, the girls with autism who were somewhat included and involved start to drift more and more to the outskirts. Most of them struggle to keep up with the fast pace of interchanges of female relationships—the chatting about boys, or gossiping about other girls.

~

Your child likely wants friends—it's a misconception that all people with ASD are antisocial. If they are rebuffed, over time they will learn to avoid social interactions in order to protect themselves from pain. Make certain your child is taught how to navigate friendship. The rules for social interaction change with age, so you'll need to stay on top of it.

~

Keep yourself in a happy place. Easier said than done many times, I know. But your emotions have significant repercussions on your daughter, which should serve as a reminder and motive to keep things as positive as possible. Eliminate all negative influences, thoughts, and people if necessary. You and your daughter don't have time for negativity!

~

Dealing with emotions is one of the more difficult areas for kids on the spectrum. One strategy you can follow is when your child gets emotional remember to "label" the emotion for him or her. Giving them a description of how they are feeling will help them to understand, learn and manage their feelings. This can be particularly useful in battling tantrums; just remember to work on the feelings after the child has calmed. You can use PECS or other visuals to describe the emotions if the child is non-verbal.

Encourage Your Child to Succeed: Building Self-Esteem

Raise your daughter to have good self-esteem, a necessary trait for a successful life. This means raising her with the firm knowledge that you love her and believe in her. Set high expectations for your girl, but give her the means to reach them. Teach her that she has the right to her own opinion, and respect the choices she makes when she is given the opportunity to choose. Raise her to believe that with hard work, she can reach her goals. In this way, she can reach her true potential.

—Chantal Sicile-Kira, www.chantalsicile-kira.com

~

Dads, the great thing about your ASD daughter is that she may be more likely to want to help you fix the car and build a fort than help Mom cook dinner. This is a trait that may be overlooked because she's "in her head" and so solitary much of the time.

—Rudy Simone, *Aspergirls*

~

Girls with autism tend to have interests that are more typically identified as boy interests than girl interests. They may be more interested in figuring out how to build a working backyard rocket than in playing with dolls. It's important to encourage their natural abilities and give them positive feedback for pursuing their area of interest.

~

Parents should not allow autism to define their child. Just as one would not narrowly define a child with high blood sugar by saying "My child is diabetes," a child with autistic features and manifestations should not be labeled "autism." Your child is not autism. Your child is a sweet and wonderful individual who, just like all of us, has multiple positive attributes and a variety of challenges that need to be addressed.

—Dr. Mark Freilich, Total Kids Developmental
Pediatric Resources, New York City

~

Many children with autism are good at drawing, art, and computer programming. These talent areas should be encouraged. I think there needs to be much more emphasis on developing the child's talents. Talents can be turned into skills that can be used for future employment.

—Temple Grandin, PhD, author of
Thinking in Pictures and *The Way I See It*,
www.autism.com/ind_teaching_tips.asp

~

As much as possible, treat your children as though they were typically developing. Kids will always live up to your lowest expectations.

—Judith chinitz, MS, MS, CNC, author of *We Band of Mothers*

~

Overly focusing on a child as if they are a problem to solve in order to be happy creates self-esteem issues. Resist this! Also, encouraging independence at each stage of development, even before the child seems ready, usually pays off in more success and stronger self-esteem.

—Lynette Louise, MS, Board certified in Neurofeedback by BCIA, NTCB

~

Go out in the community. Don't close your child in at home. Take your child to amusement parks, the zoo, or to visit friends and relatives.

Making Sure Your Child Gets to Be a Kid

Let your child be involved in picking an activity or two each week. Give her the responsibility of coming up with something that interests her and involves a trip away from the home.

Responding to Undesirable Behavior

Just because your child has autism is no reason to steer clear of consequences for bad behavior. As with any typical child, she will smell weakness and take advantage if you let her get away with misbehavior.

~

Children with autism respond differently to sensory input. Some enjoy or crave constant input while others become agitated by it. And some children will respond differently depending on the day, time, or situation. Undesirable behavior is often a result of a child's reaction to sensory input. Observe her closely in order to determine what stimuli negatively affect her behavior.

~

Keep your behaviors in check. We are all prone to overreaction on occasion and these potentially intense outbursts (either positive or negative) can confuse and dysregulate your daughter. Keeping an even keel should be your focus.

~

Don't threaten a punishment you're not prepared to enforce. If you're not really going to cancel the birthday party, don't say you will. Don't count to three or ten—your child will learn that she always has that long, and you didn't mean it the first time. If you teach a two-year-old, gently, but firmly, that you mean what you say, you don't have to keep teaching it—at sixteen, she will still know that you meant it the first time. Too often parents allow their children to push them around because they want to be liked, but your child will neither like nor respect you. Children crave boundaries.

Managing Severe Aggression

Tips by Cathy Purple Cherry, AIA, LEED AP

Our ASD son was physically aggressive from the age of fourteen through now at the age of nineteen. His aggression was mostly displayed passively and through self-mutilation. On occasion, it was quite violent and sometimes directed towards his siblings. He has put his head and foot through a wall several times and punched himself to create blood and then bled all over the floor. Most recently, he attempted to stab himself with a big stick. My tips come from these past five years.

- The hardest lesson I had to teach myself was that an audience made the aggressive behavior of our ASD child worse. So, I learned to walk away, close the door, turn off the light and ignore. It took me at least three years to get to this place.

- Prevention is possible in some cases especially when it comes to reducing conflict between the ASD child and their siblings. Violation of personal space is a major trigger. Thus, prevent path crossing and entering of each others' rooms. I would orchestrate all the time which direction around the furniture I wanted my ASD son to travel so he would not run into his brother or sister.

- My son was famous for full body dropping as a negative and passive aggressive response. After he had self-mutilated, he would drop and shut down with no response whatsoever. I called these his "fits" . . . and there weren't five in his life but rather maybe four hundred. If he was not in his own bedroom and, if I could, I removed him from our home and placed him on the grass in the yard. I watched from inside the house but absolutely did not let him know I was watching. Autistic children need time to learn to overcome their "fight" response.

- If your ASD child is violent, take him to the emergency ward at your hospital to have him temporarily committed to a psych hospital or call the police. Remove the threat from your home and inform others of what is happening.

- Medication changes can, at times, help. Do not hide these behaviors from your support team. Communicate immediately with your child's psychiatrist. Also, be aware that there is a calming medication that can be given just before these explosive episodes if you can see them coming. Again, speak with your child's psychiatrist.

Working with Your Partner or Spouse

The following tips are adapted from an article by Toni Schutta, MA, LP, Parent Coach, author, and founder of www.getparentinghelpnow.com.

Reach an agreement to support each other publicly (or at least to remain neutral). You've heard about the importance of presenting a united front so your child can't divide and conquer, and it's true. It's confusing to your child when you argue about consequences in front of them. Children with a manipulative nature will use the situation to their advantage. Usually what happens is that you get embroiled in your own debate and the disciplinary action gets forgotten. It also undermines your spouse's parental authority in front of your child, which is something you don't want to do.

~

Develop a signal. Let's say that you strongly disagree with the other parent's choice of discipline. Agree ahead of time on a signal that you can give that means, "Take a break. let's talk about this." Perhaps making a "T" sign with your hands to signal a time-out would be a good choice.

~

Talk privately about the child's offense and how it should be handled. There are few disciplinary actions that can't wait for a few minutes. Taking the time to leave the room and talk privately with your spouse about how to handle the situation is a respectful way of communicating to your spouse that there might be other options to consider. Regardless, you are setting a much-needed boundary that this is an adult matter, and that the two of you will handle it accordingly, as a team.

~

Check in with the other parent to see if they've already made a decision. Many children will use the one-liner "Dad said that I could" to get what they want. When hearing this line from your child, a wise thing to do is to actually ask the other parent if she has already given approval to your child's request. Again, this demonstrates to your child that as parents, you are united and will support each other. Usually your child starts backpedaling if she is trying to manipulate you.

~

Develop three to four consistent family rules for the most common misbehaviors. For instance, all families should have a rule that "no one's body will be hurt by hitting, kicking, biting, etc." Consistent discipline should be applied by both parents when physical aggression occurs. Parents will never agree on how to handle all offenses, but if parents respond consistently to the top three behaviors, it will make a significant impact.

~

Agree that smaller offenses can be handled at the discretion of the parent in charge. Once you have your family rules in place, try not to sweat the small stuff. It can be beneficial for children to learn different methods of problem-solving and communication, so if your spouse parents a little differently, it might actually benefit your child. For instance, some parents are better at using humor to move through tough situations, and if you're open to it, you can learn what works more effectively with each child.

Don't blame the other adult. No one is to "blame" for the child's problems. Enlist the strengths of each member of the family, anyone who can help.

—Stanley I. Greenspan, MD, *The Supportive Family Environment*

Defusing the Meltdown from Hell

When your daughter is having a meltdown, try to remove others from the situation before trying to move the dysregulated child. It could help prevent the situation from escalating.

—Megan Miller, Head Teacher

~

Practice deep breathing to help you stay calm during stressful times with your child. The calmer you are, the safer your child will feel, which can help prevent meltdowns from escalating even more.

—Jenn Gross, OTR/L

~

Set up a safe, small, quiet space that your child can use during times of frustration and anger. This gives them a comforting place of their own where they can retreat when they need a break.

—Jenn Gross, OTR/L

~

Ice: When battling the meltdown from hell, deploy ice! Chewing and holding ice can help calm your daughter down. She can also help in the creation and storage of ice in the freezer, giving her a reference point. Many kids will seek out a particular sensory input when on the verge of melting down; ice can serve as one more tool to help them self regulate. So remember, when in hell, freeze it over!

~

Anything added to systems already struggling to create and maintain stability can be overwhelming. "Anything" can mean perfumes, crowds (especially of children), household cleaning products, and even medications. Behavioral expectations beyond the person's ability are problematic.

—Carolyn Nuyens and Marlene Suliteanu, "The Holistic Approach to Neurodevelopment and Learning Efficiency (HANDLE)," *Cutting-Edge Therapies for Autism*

~

Productive Approaches to Parenting

A "tantrum" or "meltdown" is actually a call for help, a plea to notice that the stress level has overflowed its container. A word of caution to family members: Try to identify what pushed your loved one beyond endurance—and don't expect it to always be the same thing. It could be noise in high-ceilinged supermarkets, or maybe it was the crowds, or smells, or any combination of these things. Always trust that there is a precipitating cause.

—Carolyn Nuyens and Marlene Suliteanu,
"The Holistic Approach to Neurodevelopment
and Learning Efficiency (HANDLE),"
Cutting-Edge Therapies for Autism

~

Parents should work with schools in this regard, too; some children use this behavior as a way to get out of class or sent home, and if the school removes them, it just shows them they can get their way.

~

Parents must carefully evaluate their response patterns to be consistent with regard to problematic behavior.

—Jenifer Clark, MA, PhD(c), "Applied Behavior Analysis,"
Cutting-Edge Therapies for Autism

~

I have already mentioned the importance of keeping a journal or diary and provided a sample worksheet (www.

skyhorsepublishing.com/Therapy_logbook.xls) to do so.
Here is another use for that log—analyzing the meltdown.
If you note diet, time of year, day, weather, and such in this
log and track meltdowns, you may uncover a pattern that
can then be broken or at least prepared for. You may be able
to preempt many a meltdown with the patterns you notice.

~

Never try to teach during a meltdown. It won't work.
Ask yourself how open you are to learning when you are
angry, terrified, overwrought, overanxious, or otherwise
emotionally disabled.

—Ellen Notbohm and Veronica Zysk,
1001 Great Ideas for Teaching and
Raising Children with Autism Spectrum Disorders

~

When you sense a tantrum developing, shift gears and work
to redirect your child's focus. Keep handy chewy toys, ice,
or a favorite video, which may help nip a meltdown in the
bud. Teach all your child's caregivers the warning signs and
share strategies with them and other parents.

~

Ignore the tantrum. Seriously—this can work. Of course,
it can only be applied at home. You could ignore a tantrum
once you've brought her home from an off-site meltdown.
A frustration meltdown has the best synergy with this
strategy, as she will likely move on to something else, or

just run out of steam. Then you can follow up with some queries as to what happened and try to understand what you can do to avoid this next time.

~

During meltdowns, work to keep everybody safe. At home you can have some strategies in place. When out in the community, this can become difficult and potentially drag others into it; it's best to remove your child from the location as quickly as possible.

~

Tantrums may scare you in their intensity, but they are typically a cry for help or understanding or even pain. It is a communication issue and your child is as afraid as you.

CHAPTER 7
Personal Care

Toileting Skills

Toileting was typically difficult for us. Without using their names to preserve their privacy a bit, I'll tell you what worked for each of my daughters. Oh, and what do I consider "toilet trained?" The day I did not see pee or poop that had not come out of my OWN body was the day the girl was fully trained. That said, none of my girls wipe their bottoms sufficiently, so there's still work to do.

One daughter was trained by a wonderful school paraprofessional who sat my daughter on the toilet, listened to her shriek at the top of her lungs, and kept her on the toilet until she peed there. After two or three successes, my daughter lost her fear and was pretty much trained. It took tough love. And ear plugs. We still pray for Mrs. D in our prayers.

One daughter used to poop standing up at her computer. We tried everything to get her to go on the toilet, including moving the computer (a wired desktop!) into the bathroom, table and all. Nope. She would not go while seated. We worked with her diet and used stool softeners to help her. One day, I went into the bathroom and there was poop. I recognized it as hers. (That doesn't faze you, does it?) She went in the toilet in her own sweet time. She was almost twelve.

One daughter presented a bigger challenge than her darling sisters. She did not use the toilet to pee or poop but she sure loved the toilet! If you've read my memoir you know I have a chapter called "Crapisode." After several bathroom floods *avec merde*, I had to call on a professional. I was at the National Autism Conference and met Brenda Batts, autism Mom and author of *Ready, Set, Potty* from Jessica Kingsley Publishing. I followed her advice for girls exactly and it worked!

~

Tips by Cathy Purple Cherry, AIA, LEED AP
Children with autism often learn through constantly repeated routines. Thus, the solution to successful toilet training may be tied to repeated practice. Be diligent. When you look back on the many years of rearing an ASD child to adulthood, you will realize "patience" was your child's gift to you! Thus, practice and patience, practice and patience, practice and patience, multiplied hundreds of times.

~

An ASD child is not always aware of her surroundings. Their tactile sensitivities can be somewhat dulled. Our son is minimally affected by heat and cold, for example. Thus, recognize that the child may not care if she has made a mess in her clothing. Acceptance by you of this behavior may be the bigger challenge and the only solution.

~

A reward system is known to be successful at school for modifying behaviors. Try a point sheet or rewards chart that leads to something good if your child takes steps towards successful toilet training. For our son, during a time in his development, a can of cherry pie filling was more motivating to him that an ice cream sundae so play to the interests at the time!

~

Develop a silent signal between you and your daughter so that she can quietly communicate her bathroom urges to you before accidents happen. If she uses this signal, reward her.

For children with autism, toilet training often occurs at only slightly later than expected ages for typically developing children . . . For more moderately to severely impaired children, a good rule of thumb is to wait until non-language mental age is in the eighteen- to twenty-four-month age range.

—Bryna Siegel, *Helping Children with Autism Learn*

If you are having problems with nighttime wettings, you may need to increase the frequency of bathroom visits. Set your alarm for every hour or two and bring her to the bathroom even if she appears to not have to go. As you get drier nights extend the time between visits until you are all good for the evening. Do not get discouraged by the occasional backslide. With any luck, she'll eventually be able to make it through the night.

~

FYI: some meds, most notably risperidone/risperdal, have the side effect of lessening urination control. Check your meds and review side effects.

—Lynette Louise, MS, Board certified in Neurofeedback by BCIA, NTCB

~

Some children might also want to have flushable wet wipes available to improve their after-toilet cleanup, and thereby avoid dirtying their clothes. Wipes can be purchased in small, discreet containers that fit well in a purse or backpack.

—*Autistic Spectrum Disorders: Understanding the Diagnosis & Getting Help* by Mitzi Waltz. Published by O'Reilly Media, Inc. Copyright © 2002 Mitzi Waltz. All rights reserved. Used with permission. http://oreilly.com/medical/autism/news/tips_life.html

~

A common problem is that a child might be able to use the toilet correctly at home but refuse to use it at school. This might be due to a failure to recognize the toilet. Hilde De Clercq from Belgium discovered that an autistic child might use a small non-relevant detail to recognize an object such as a toilet. It takes detective work to find that detail. In one case a boy would only use the toilet at home that had a black seat. His parents and teacher were able to get him to use the toilet at school by covering its white seat with black tape. The tape was then gradually removed and toilets with white seats became recognized as toilets.

—Temple Grandin, PhD, author of
Thinking in Pictures and *The Way I See It*,
www.autism.com/ind_teaching_tips.asp

~

If bedwetting remains an issue, rule out allergic bedwetting. If nighttime soiling is a problem, consult a knowledgeable gastroenterologist who has experience with children with autism. This might be a symptom of a gastrointestinal disorder.

Bathing Skills

My daughters' middle school teacher made a cassette tape with a shower song, using "This is the way we wash our feet . . ." and then all of the body parts, up to the hair. By turning on the tape player during shower time, my girls were able to wash their own bodies with the music as a reminder.

~

One of my girls used to pour her shampoo into her hand, and while recapping the bottle, all of the shampoo would rinse off her hand and down the drain. Purchase a shampoo dispenser that is easy to use to ensure clean hair.

~

Parents have a powerful weapon in their fight against autism: water. The bathtub, shower, or pool can offer countless opportunities to tame transitional stresses, promote social encounters, correct out-of-kilter motor systems, and promote sensory integration.

—Andrea Salzman, "Aquatic Therapy,"
Cutting-Edge Therapies for Autism

~

Parents who are greeted with unceasing crying jags every evening at bath time can try this trick for co-bathing. Take a towel, swaddle the child, offer the child the bottle, and then lower the child into a warm bath cradled in your arms. This works best if the child can be handed to an already-positioned parent ready in the tub. The transition is smoothed by the act of swaddling, immersion in skin-temperature water, and positioning in the cradling/nursing position. Yet, the child is successfully making a transition. Over time, the props can be removed and the transition can become more dramatic.

—Andrea Salzman, "Aquatic Therapy,"
Cutting-Edge Therapies for Autism

~

Even for older kids, tub toys, soap "paints," bubble bath, or other items might allow you to get them in and out of a warm tub once a week.

~

Contrary to popular belief, it's not necessary to bathe children daily unless there are special medical or sanitary reasons to do so. Use a washcloth to zap any particularly grungy areas daily, and schedule an unavoidable bath time for one or more days each week. A flexible shower hose can be very useful for washing the hair of children who are afraid of the big shower.

Dental Hygiene at Home

Be persistent with toothbrushing, even if it is difficult. Be sure to make brushing teeth a routine part of your child's routine, morning and night. Start by counting to ten slowly while brushing so that your child knows when it will be over. Gradually add more time so that you are able to brush the entire mouth well.

—Ruby Gelman, DMD

~

Water is a great help to keep the mouth clean after meals. Drinking a few ounces of water after a meal can significantly reduce the acid buildup that begins with chewing and swallowing food. This can be a great help in preventing cavities.

—Ruby Gelman, DMD

~

Given our kids' sensory issues, you may have a tough time finding an acceptable toothbrush. Luckily nowadays there are many to try! Experiment with different bristles, head sizes, and those that vibrate. We have had success with the Oral-B battery-operated brushes; they make it a bit more fun and have the added benefit of being more effective.

~

When brushing your child's teeth, experiment with different brushing angles in order to be not only effective, but also comfortable enough from a sensory standpoint. Likewise, try different pastes and gels to get the right flavor and texture.

Haircuts

~

If you can figure out what it is about haircuts that drives your child wild, then remove that particular trigger. You may then be able to get the job done at a regular barbershop or salon, with modifications. Common problems and solutions include:

- Sensitivity to barbershop or salon odors: if this is the case, look for an old-fashioned barbershop that eschews smelly shampoos, or buy a home hair-cutting kit. Unscented products are often available, but you may have to buy them yourself and bring them in, or request them in advance.

- Sensitivity to the sound of buzzing clippers or snapping scissors: some people can tolerate one but not the other. There are also old-fashioned hand razors for cutting hair, but it's hard to find a barber who can wield one with precision. Call around! You might also try earplugs, or an iPod playing a favorite song through

> headphones. Your barber will happily work
> around headphones if it keeps the child in the
> chair. You might also choose to accept a longer
> hairstyle, if grooming is not a problem.

Some places will be flexible; it might help to go outside
of usual business hours. Some that cater to children have
DVD players. A massage during the cut can do wonders.

Personal Hygiene

Body odors: Teach your girls to change into fresh
underwear both at bedtime and in the morning. This helps
keep the body fresh and avoid odors.

Love's Baby Soft is an old perfume that is still available.
I allow my teen girls to wear it to help them remain fresh-
smelling throughout the day. Its soft, powdery scent is
appropriate and pleasant.

~

Most girls with autism do not learn what they need to
know independently about hygiene and health, and this
is an area that must be emphasized. Sometimes the lack
of implementing has to do with the girl having trouble
remembering the steps or which routine to do when, and
sometimes it is due to a lack of motor planning ability.

~

Some girls like to wear the same thing over and over because of the feel of the fabric or the image on the shirt. This becomes unacceptable as they get older. Tell her these clothes can be worn at home, in private (i.e., not when special guests are over). Find some comfortable replacements that are appropriate for her age for her to wear out of the house.

~

It's important to find a teen peer to go shopping with your daughter. You may think you know what is cool or "in," but a peer knows intuitively what the girls are wearing and what your daughter should wear. Looking like they fit in is really helpful, and encourages success in social situations with peers.

~

Good hygiene needs to be addressed in girls early on, and good habits developed and emphasized. Explain why it's important (social stories tailored to ability level). There are health reasons (we need to do this to stay healthy) and there are social reasons (we need to stay clean in order to make friends).

~

Using visual supports (including modeling) can be the most effective strategy when teaching about hygiene and grooming. For shaving legs, you might attach a laminated card to the bathtub detailing the different steps (according to her needs), including reminders for steps she sometimes forgets along with pictures of each step.

—Shana Nichols, Gina Marie Moravcik,
and Samara Pulver Tetenbaum,
Girls Growing Up on the Autism Spectrum

~

Many AS girls think that spending a lot of money and time on their appearance is illogical and stupid, but if they think of it as the "uniform" to getting the job (i.e., the relationship), then they might be more inclined to put it on.

—Rudy Simone, *Aspergirls*

Clothing

The following tips are adapted from *Autistic Spectrum Disorders: Understanding the Diagnosis & Getting Help* by Mitzi Waltz. Published by O'Reilly Media, Inc. Copyright © 2002 Mitzi Waltz. All rights reserved. Used with permission. http://oreilly.com/medical/autism/news/tips_life.html

• What do you do with a child who strips off her clothes at every opportunity? First, you try to find out why. The most common reason is sensory sensitivity, so first talk to an occupational therapist about instituting a program of sensory integration therapy. In the meantime, see what you can do to make staying clothed more comfortable. Verbal children may be able to explain what they don't like about wearing clothes. Common problems include chafing waistbands, itchy fabrics, "new-clothes" smell, and annoying tags. Kids who can't stand regular waistbands can often handle elastic-waist pants and shorts, especially those made with soft fabrics, such as sweatpants. Others can wear only overalls or coveralls with ease, and these have the added "bonus" of being harder to remove.

- For children who wear diapers, the diaper itself may be the problem. Check for and treat any actual diaper rash. (Incidentally, diaper rash can be caused by a yeast infection on the skin, which may indicate a larger problem with yeast overgrowth.) Experiment with different types of cloth diapers, various brands of disposables, and larger diapers if tightness around the waist and legs is an issue.

- Over-the-diaper or training pants, sweatpants, overalls (especially the ones with snaps along the inseam), coveralls, and jumpsuits all work well. Some parents actually stitch down the overall straps each morning, or replace easy-open fasteners with something more complex. It's possible to open overalls and coveralls for larger children along the inseam and add unobtrusive snaps or Velcro for easy toileting without complete clothes removal.

- Shirts and dresses that button up the back are also hard to remove.

- Explore catalogs that carry special clothing for children with disabilities. Many items in these catalogs are especially good for older children who have toileting problems, or for children with orthopedic impairments in addition to an ASD.

- Many people with sensory problems prefer soft fabrics, such as cotton jersey or terrycloth, over stiff fabrics like denim. If this is the case with your child, go shopping with that in mind. It can help to wash new clothing a few times before wearing it, to remove that stiff feeling as well as any unfamiliar smells. [Alternatively, some children complain that very soft fabrics feel "like dust."]

- If an aversion to clothing crops up suddenly, make sure you haven't just changed your detergent or fabric softener. There may be a smell or allergy issue going on.

- Remove tags from inside of garments as needed.

- One solution that will save you money and hassles is purchasing used clothing instead of new ones. These pre-softened garments may already feel "just right." Again, they may need to be washed a few times to take away any bothersome scents.

Here is a "bra ladder" you can use to prepare your daughter for wearing a full-fledged bra:

- Loose tank top or camisole
- Fitted tank top or camisole (e.g., with a built-in shelf bra)
- Training bra
- Sports bra
- Soft cup bra
- Underwire bra

—Shana Nichols, Gina Marie Moravcik,
and Samara Pulver Tetenbaum,
Girls Growing Up on the Autism Spectrum

Puberty

Girls who do not like change may get upset when they see their body beginning to change and grow differently, and they realize they have no control over it. Explaining that everyone's body changes, and showing baby, children, teen, and current photos of adult family members will help them understand that puberty and growing happens to everyone.

~

Make sure to use correct names of body parts (i.e., breasts, vagina), but also teach the synonyms that they may hear from others (i.e., boobs).

~

Explain that good and bad feelings will come as part of changing into an adult body. Girls who are interested in logic and facts may be interested in charting their own moods on a calendar to see if there is a cyclical pattern coinciding with their menstrual cycle.

~

Have a collection of ideas to help adolescent girls when their mood is low (remember risk of depression). What activities can they do, what music can they listen to, that will make them feel happier?

~

Explain that some changes will only be associated with the same sex (e.g., a boy will not begin to grow breasts, but a girl will), and this needs to be explained to both boys and girls. Explain that hair will only grow in certain places (the child may think the whole body eventually becomes progressively covered in hair, like a werewolf). Explain that extra hair just grows on the underarms and on the pubic area in women. Explain that on men, extra hair grows on the underarms and on the pubic area, and on the chest, face, and chin.

~

Make sure that when your daughter is going through puberty, you take her to her doctor for all necessary examinations and assessments, to ensure (as for any teen girl) that all is progressing as it should be.

~

One out of four teens with autism is at risk of developing seizure activity during their adolescent years, possibly due to hormonal changes in the body. The seizures may be associated with convulsions, and others may be minor and not detected by simple observation.

~

When girls reach puberty and start showing more noncompliant behaviors, many parents think "oh no—her autism is getting worse!" Actually, noncompliance is normal teenage behavior. At this point, parents need to remember to give the teen more choices in which to express herself and to have more control over some aspects of her day, within defined limits.

~

Precocious puberty has been estimated to be twenty times higher in children with neurodevelopmental disabilities, including autism.

~

It is important to begin teaching girls about their changing bodies before they hit puberty. Teaching them about the changes that will occur in the boy's body as well as their own body is important. Otherwise, they may be surprised by the changes they see in their male classmates, and not understand why they look different if they have not seen them for some time (i.e., summer vacation).

~

Girls usually start puberty before boys, at around the age of eight or nine. In girls, overall body shape starts to change as breasts and hips begin to develop. Often they have pubic hair by the time they are ten or eleven. Their first period may arrive between the ages of eleven and twelve; however, girls do develop at different rates, so it is difficult to predict for sure.

~

Puberty can be a difficult time for a girl on the spectrum, as usually they like predictability and routine, and many have a difficult time with change. Many have a hard time with the fact that their body is growing and changing and there is nothing they can do to stop it.

~

Drugs and alcohol: alcoholic drinks or drugs often react adversely with your child's prescriptions, so you have to teach your teen girl about these dangers. If your daughter is very rule-oriented, try emphasizing that drugs and alcohol are illegal.

—www.yourlittleprofessor.com/teen2.html

~

To prepare your daughter for her first pelvic exam, have your daughter be present for one of your pelvic exams (or another family member's); schedule a pre-exam appointment, in which only parts of the full examination are conducted and the rest are explained; or create a picture story for her.

—Shana Nichols, Gina Marie Moravcik,
and Samara Pulver Tetenbaum,
Girls Growing Up on the Autism Spectrum

~

The emotional instability and moodiness of adolescent girls can be amplified for girls with ASD as estrogen begins to impact them. Additional social-emotional goals to be considered at this time include identifying a variety of emotions, recognizing signs of stress, utilizing stress management tools, and staying calm during stressful periods.

—Lori Ernsperger, PhD, and Danielle Wendel,
Girls Under the Umbrella of Autism Spectrum Disorders

Periods

How many of you flipped straight to this part of the book? Menstruation is a panic-inducing topic for us. Of all the milestones our girls might miss, why do they have to reach this one? The rite of passage into womanhood signals that time is slipping away from us. Our girls are growing up. The psychological impact can really get under our skin. Periods mean pregnancy is a possibility. Pregnancy means sex. Some of our girls might experience a loving sex life with a partner. Some might never know the closeness and pleasure of lovemaking. Then there's the "not going there" topic of assault. Periods bring all of these musings into sharp focus for Moms and Dads alike. I can't help much with the fear, but the tips below can help you prepare yourself, your male partner, and your daughter.

My daughters got their periods at nine and a half, eleven, and thirteen. We used pads and only pads at this time. One summer, I was juggling the "can we go swimming?" calendar and a good friend with a typical daughter said, "Why don't you just give them tampons?" I explained that in my girls' black-and-white world, it's safer to have a rule that nothing goes into their bodies. My friend understood immediately, but was surprised. "I've never thought of that."

~

Periods throw our body chemistry into turmoil. Some "aspergirls" don't really show strong autistic symptoms until puberty. Prior to this we may just seem gifted; but when puberty hits, it flips us on our heads and you can see our autistic underbelly.

—Rudy Simone, *Aspergirls*

~

Not all girls are physically or cognitively able to self-manage their menstruation cycle. But you never know till you try. By teaching as much as possible, as often as possible, many girls can surpass expectations that are set. It is important to give them the benefit of the doubt to increase their independence.

~

Talk to your girl about her changing body using social stories and/or images, in simple terms. It is important to start explaining before they begin menstruating so they are not surprised. Fourth grade is usually a good time to begin this conversation. Explain what periods are, what purpose they serve, how often they occur, and what to do about them.

~

Using a matter-of-fact attitude and voice when discussing menstruation is best. Even if the girl is nonverbal, assume she under-stands and go over the information many times, over a period of time.

~

If the girl has sensory issues, it is a good idea to have her practice wearing a sanitary pad before she begins to menstruate in order to help her get used to the feel of the pad against her body. The girl may need to wear it for short periods of time, adding more time as she gets used to the pad. This way, when she begins to menstruate, she will not have to deal with the new feel of the pad as well as the blood flow.

~

Girls must be told that talking about periods and cramps is "private" conversation, meaning something you talk about in private. Private means at home with your close family. They need to learn it's not appropriate to talk about in a public setting (i.e., during lunchtime in the school cafeteria).

~

Creating a set of photo sequence cards with step-by-step instructions on how to change sanitary pads is helpful for many. Going over it and practicing before a girl begins to menstruate will help ward off any fears.

~

For school, having a bathroom folder that a girl takes with her to the bathroom (along with the necessary sanitary pad) will remind her of the steps to be taken, including the all-important part of washing hands.

~

Girls need to be taught about menstruation and the fact that they will be experiencing a flow of blood on a regular basis, before they begin to menstruate. Otherwise, they may think there is something very wrong when their first menses appear.

~

A mother of a daughter with autism shared with me how her daughter learned where to place her menstrual pad. The mom traced an outline of the pad on the underwear so the daughter could independently place the pad into the shape that was traced. This way, the pad was put in the correct place and she could avoid any accidents that might occur if the pad was placed too high or too low on her underwear.

—Bonnie Waring, LMSW

~

Exchange diapers for panties with mini pads and talk about being a big girl. Bring your child into your inner circle so she is privy to how you put on a pad (tampons are too intrusive and scary) and how you clean yourself. It is always best to treat these issues in a matter-of-fact way. "Mommy wears this to keep her bottom clean if she leaks." As your daughter grows, talk to her in an age-appropriate way, teaching "as if" she understands. Then guide her along, believing that even though she may understand, she will still need lots of repetition.

—Lynette Louise, MS, Board certified
in Neurofeedback by BCIA, NTCB

~

Have your daughter practice using the thinnest menstrual pads you can find (without wings—they are too sticky) at the first sign of breast buds or underarm hair. She'll need to become accustomed to the sensation of the pad, and to practice placement and removal in a sanitary way, long before her first period arrives. Teach the skill before she needs it to cut down on stress for both mom and daughter. And teach Dad, too; he's going to have to know how to help his daughter when Mom is not around.

~

Using a drawing of her reproductive system, illustrate how an egg is released from the ovary, travels down the fallopian tube, and eventually sits in the wall of the uterus. Use a red crayon to demonstrate how the uterine lining becomes thicker as the egg gets closer to the uterus.

> —Shana Nichols, Gina Marie Moravcik,
> and Samara Pulver Tetenbaum,
> *Girls Growing Up on the Autism Spectrum*

~

Make a social storybook and read it quite often. If your daughter has a Dynavox, make another story for that, explaining what to expect and why. Make a "period box." In it, put pads, Advil, and personal wipes. Keep it in her room. When the moment arrives, go straight to the box. If possible, celebrate this important rite of passage. Try to make the situation positive instead of negative.

> —Kathy Hudson, Mom to Abby

~

Keep feminine hygiene products in every bathroom and a set in the glove box of your car, in case your child's period appears unexpectedly. Early on, periods will be unpredictable.

Masturbation

If your daughter starts to rub often around her vagina, she may be starting to explore masturbation, but she may also be experiencing itching due to yeast infection. Parents need to make sure their teenage girl has necessary exams to rule out any medical concerns.

Masturbation is normal teenage activity; however, most teenagers know to masturbate in private. Not so for girls on the spectrum. Parents need to teach their teenage girls the concept of private and public, and that masturbation is a private activity, not a public one.

~

Touching in the genital area should be addressed as soon as it shows up regardless of age or gender. Just say matter-of-factly: "Touching your penis (or vulva) is for private time. Please wait till you are in bed at night." There is no room for emotions here. If you are vague or nervous, your child will likely continue to grow more inappropriate. Be clear and nonjudgmental. It works well.

—Lynette Louise, MS, Board certified
in Neurofeedback by BCIA, NTCB

Sexuality and Sex Education

Don't be afraid to address sexuality and sexual behavior with children and adolescents who have autism, as they have the same basic human needs like everyone else. Failure to address this subject matter can lead to confusion, inappropriate behavior, and/or things that can be both physically and emotionally damaging. Start educating children with autism about their sexuality early on. It is most beneficial when the information comes from their parent/caregiver.

—Dr. Mary Jo Lang

~

If the teenage girl is physically mature but delayed socially and emotionally, but is also gregarious, communicate openly and consistently with the girl's teachers, care providers, and, if appropriate, with local authorities, on where the girl is at in development, as well as what you are teaching them. This will help prevent social and/or legal issues arising from any possible inappropriate public behavior.

~

Teach your daughter early and often the basics about sexual awareness: what is sex, what is acceptable behavior, and when is it acceptable? Teach about boundaries: what boundaries should we have for our bodies, as well as when interacting with others?

~

If your daughter sits in on sex education classes offered at the school for the mainstream population, she may hear all the facts but not personalize the information and realize that it is meant for her. This means that as a parent, you will need to verify that she has understood how this information relates to her.

~

Address self-protection skills that encourage children and adolescents with autism to say "no" and to avoid individuals who seek to take advantage of them. It has been reported that children with disabilities are 2.2 times more likely to be sexually abused, making self-protection skills important to address and develop.

—Dr. Mary Jo Lang

Chapter 8

Safety

Personal Safety

Teaching the concept of "private" to little girls will help them understand important rules of private vs. public behavior. As they get older, it's important to have additional conversations about the topic, to help them understand rules of personal safety. At home, teach your daughter that it is okay to have clothes off in private areas of the house (i.e., their bedroom), but that in public areas of the house (living room, kitchen, etc.), they must keep their clothes on. use picture icons if needed.

~

Girls on the spectrum need to know what constitutes sexual abuse. Nonverbal children and teens are at a high risk for sexual and physical abuse because of the perception that they are unable to communicate what happens to them. They are often grouped in classrooms or camp situations where predators know they can find victims.

~

Girls on the more able end of the spectrum are at high risk for sexual abuse because they are not good at figuring out people's intentions (i.e., picking up on nonverbal cues). This is why it's important for them to be taught what constitutes a sexual act and what is appropriate and inappropriate behavior.

~

It is important for the girl's safety that she be able to identify places on her body where it is appropriate to be touched by others. It is important that the girl be able to communicate to someone when she has been touched in an "off-limits" area on her body. Off-limits areas of the body are those normally covered by a bathing suit.

~

Teach your girl how to say "no" emphatically, and to mean it. For those with little verbal skills, teach them how to clearly show they do not want the person to come any closer.

~

Girls need to learn what sex is, and what constitutes a sex act. Girls with Asperger's and on the more able end of the spectrum are more apt to be victimized by others because of their gullibility. If they know what constitutes a sex act (including oral sex), and they understand about when it is appropriate or not to engage in sexual acts, they are less likely to be victimized.

Home Safety

Stove safety is a big issue, and tiny plastic shields do not help when you have a child who is curious and taller than the stove. For those with children who simply will not leave it alone, you can go so far as to install the expensive but fully effective ($400) stove guard machine that disables the stove unless the right password is entered. Obviously this is not the solution for everyone, but if your child has a history of dangerously playing with the stove, it might be worth it.

—Candi Summers, Autism & Parenting Examiner,
examiner.com, http://exm.nr/9sfVh8

~

For the sneaky eater you can install a padlock on the fridge door or chain locks on cabinets. You can also put medicine and cleaning supplies inside a locked cabinet with a Tot lok on it.

—Candi Summers, Autism & Parenting Examiner,
examiner.com, http://exm.nr/9sfVh8

Runners

The following tips are adapted from *Autistic Spectrum Disorders: Understanding the Diagnosis & Getting Help* by Mitzi Waltz. Published by O'Reilly Media, Inc. Copyright © 2002 Mitzi Waltz. All rights reserved. Used with permission. http://oreilly.com/medical/autism/ news/tips_life.html

~

If escapes are a problem for your family, please consider using the services of a professional security consultant. You may be able to get help from government developmental-delay or mental health agencies, or private agencies, to find and even pay for these services. Most people don't wish to turn their homes into fortresses, but in some cases, it's the most caring thing you can do. It could very well save a life.

~

Double- or triple-bolt security doors can slow down a would-be escapee, and some types can be unlocked only from the inside with a key. While expensive, they are tremendously jimmy-proof. Keep the keys well hidden, of course—on your person, if need be. Fire regulations may require that an exterior-lock key be secured in a fire-box or stored at the nearest fire station in case of emergency.

~

Alarms are available that will warn you if a nocturnal roamer is approaching a door or window. Other types only sound when the door or window is actually opened. Depending on your child's speed, the latter may not give you enough response time.

~

In some cities, the local police department is sensitive to the needs and special problems of the disabled. Officers may be available to provide information about keeping your child or adult patient safe and secure, whether he lives in your home, in an institution or group home, or independently in the community. Some also have special classes to teach self-defense skills to disabled adults.

~

A few police departments also keep a registry of disabled people whose behavior could be a hazard to their own safety, or whose behavior could be misinterpreted as threatening. Avail yourself of this service if your child is an escape artist, has behaviors that could look like drunkenness or drug use to an uninformed observer, uses threatening words or gestures when afraid, or is extremely trusting of strangers.

~

People with ASDs can have a bracelet or necklace made with their home phone number, an emergency medical contact number, or the phone number of a service that can inform the caller about their diagnosis. Labels you might want to have engraved on this item include:
• Nonverbal
• Speech-impaired

- Multiple medications
- Medications include . . . (list)
- Epilepsy (or other medical condition)

~

Members of the general public, and even some safety officials, may not know the word "autistic." They are even more unlikely to know what autistic spectrum disorder (ASD) or pervasive developmental disorder (PDD) means.

There are incredible programs out there like Project lifesaver (www.projectlifesaver.org/). Project lifesaver has been commonly used with Alzheimer's patients, but has grown to address the needs of others, including those with autism, Down syndrome, traumatic brain injury, and more. People who qualify for the program are given a tracking device with a unique frequency to wear as a bracelet, which emergency responders can pick up and track with specialized equipment from one to several miles away. If your child has already gotten away from you—at home or in a public place—or you are afraid they will, see if there's a Project Lifesaver in your community and contact them. They do amazing work. There's almost always a wait list, so get on it if you qualify.

—Tim Tucker, "Practical ideas for Protecting Autistic Children before They Disappear," www.bothhandsandaflashlight.com/2010/04/16/practical-ideas-for-protecting-autistic-children-before-they-disappear/

~

Inform your neighbors about your special needs child, especially if they are a runner. Providing photos and contact information can be a lifesaver.

~

Using an alarm system, deadbolts, and window locks are necessary to secure your residence, especially if your kid is a runner.

~

Swimming is not only great exercise for your child but can serve as a safety tool as well. Frequently, kids with autism favor water and water-based activities. Keep your kid safe with some lessons!

~

If you have a runner, know where in your neighborhood your child gravitates to. These will be the likely destinations. You can also increase your frequency of visits to these locations to lessen the fascination with them.

~

Safety

As with infants, a speaker system or even a video monitor can serve to provide a level of comfort and help you transition a child into her own room.

~

Your smart phone or other device can serve to aid in tracking down a runner. Learn to use the GPS function!

~

Internal alarms: Everything depends on preventing your child from getting out in the first place. You want to build up multiple layers of "defense" against escape. If you can't stop your child from getting out of your house, slowing them down might buy you the time you need. If your child gets up and wanders around at night, install things that will either keep them in a defined area or that will notify you if they get outside that area. We have gates up around the house that are mounted directly to the wall; even most adults who visit us can't figure out how to open them. They could be hurdled by larger kids, of course. Some parents switch their child's bedroom doorknob around so it can be locked from outside the child's room. This does present a potential fire-escape hazard, though, so really think that through.

—Tim Tucker, "Practical Ideas for Protecting Autistic Children before They Disappear," www.bothhandsandaflashlight.com/2010/04/16/practical-ideas-for-protecting-autistic-children-before-they-disappear/

Car Safety

The following tips are from Tim Tucker's "Practical Ideas for Protecting Autistic Children before They Disappear," www.bothhandsandaflashlight. com/2010/04/16/practical-ideas-for-protecting-autistic-children-before- they-disappear/.

~

Especially for younger kids, escaping from their car seat can be one of the worst problems we encounter. For kids still in the five-point harness, you can simply take the lap part that everything buckles into and flip it over such that the button is facing down into the child's lap. Everything still buckles together correctly in the models I've seen. That in itself might be enough. For other kids, especially those using the regular seat belt, there are covers available that make it difficult for them to get to that release button.

~

Always enable the child locks on the rear doors of your vehicle. If adult passengers riding in your backseat complain, tell them they can walk home.

CHAPTER 9

Venturing Out

Dining Out

Your child is causing a bit of a ruckus while being out and about. A person, ignorant about autism, comments on your parenting skills and disobedient child. You walk away. Not bad, but every now and then, a rejoinder is necessary, for you (schadenfreude) and them (education) and your kid (Mom/Dad has my back!). A proven quick comeback for these times: "Sorry, she is autistic. What's your excuse?"

~

Avoid long—or, let's face it, any—restaurant waits. Go early or late to avoid any crowds. The last thing you want is a pre-meal meltdown! Try diners; we have found them to be accommodating, and they have a wide range of options.

~

Any place that has an outside seating option is great—less hassle with cleanup, and you can always take a walk.

~

Make sure the restaurant can accommodate whatever diet your child is on. This is not always easy. Google the menu and then call to confirm ingredients and how the meal you'll be ordering is prepared. Mention allergies, and make clear that MSG is off limits.

~

Once you find a good place that's suitable for your child, become a regular and tip well. In the future you'll be able to call and make special requests, or even order in advance!

~

Feel free to mention autism at the start of the meal to anyone working your table; it will help the staff understand, and you'll be able to relax.

~

Eating out provides a great opportunity for your daughter to practice self-advocacy skills, once dining out becomes possible. Teaching your daughter to ask for what she wants, and how she wants it (i.e., "I want my burger well-cooked, please." "I want ranch dressing with my fries, please." "I want the salad dressing on the side." "I want water with no ice, please."), is an enjoyable way for her to learn to speak up for herself. In this way, she will realize her opinion has an impact and is respected. As she gets older, this will help with learning to speak up for herself. Those who are nonverbal can use assistive technology to do this.

Vacations and Travel

We've taken one real family vacation. In 2007 we cashed in our Marriott points and went to Orlando for a trip to Disney. We lost Mia not once, but twice. Once on the 2000 acre property and a second time at Newark Liberty airport. And I'd prepared for everything. I had "if lost" sheets for each girl. I was on high alert. And still, Mia slipped away in the confusion and lack of routine. My advice? If you have a child who meanders, like Mia think of every safety precaution you can: tag her clothing, get a QR code in a removable tattoo or in her sneakers or on her shirt. Go to www.ifineedhelp.com for some great products and info.

~

Asking a doctor, therapist, or teacher for a letter addressed to the airline that states the child's diagnosis and challenges can cut down on wait time getting on and off a flight. Being able to hand a typed letter to someone rather than talking about your child in front of them is always a better option, especially during difficult times in the air.

—Julie Fishelson Mahan, MSW, LSW

Chantal Sicile-Kira (www.chantalsicile-kira.com) offers the following tips on travel:

Transitions are usually difficult for many on the spectrum, and traveling is really a series of transitions. Preparing the person—child, teenager, or adult—as

---

much as possible will make any trip a more enjoyable experience for all involved. Some advance planning of specific steps of the trip can be made ahead of time to prepare both the person and the environment for a better travel experience.

~

Leaving the security of home for a new place can be off-putting for individuals with autism. How you prepare the person on the spectrum depends on his or her age and ability level.

- Think of the individual's daily routine and the items she likes or needs and bring them along to make her feel more at home. Bring whatever foods and drinks will keep her happy on the trip, especially if there are dietary restrictions.

- Buy some small, inexpensive toys or books that she can play with during the journey (and if you lose them, it won't be the end of the world). if she only plays with one favorite item, try to find a duplicate and see if you can "break it in" before the trip.

- Do not wash any items (including plush toys) before the trip, as the individual may feel comfort in the "home" smell of her cherished item.

- Put up a monthly calendar with the departure date clearly marked, and have the person check off every day until departure. Bring the calendar with you and mark off the number of days in one place or on the trip, always having the return date indicated.

- Put together a picture and word "travel book" of what means of transport you are going to be using, who you are going to see, where you will sleep, and what you will do or see at your destination(s). Go over this with the person, like you would a storybook, as often as you like in preparation for the trip. Using a three-ring binder is best, as you can add extra pages or insert the calendar mentioned above for use on the trip.

- Put together a picture or word schedule of the actual journey to take with you on your trip. Add extra pages to the travel book. Add Velcro and attach pictures or words in order of the travel sequence. For example, a picture to represent the car ride to the airport, going through security, getting on the airplane, etc., for car trips, pictures representing different stops on the trip and number of miles to be driven can be used. Add an empty envelope to add the "done" pictures when you have finished one step of the journey.

- Taking a short trip before attempting longer ones is recommended, if possible. This will help the person get used to traveling and give you the opportunity to plan ahead for possible areas of difficulty. Also, if you use the travel book system, it will help the person make a connection between the travel book and any impending.

~

Some preparations can be made ahead of time for the different environments and means of transport you will be using. Most people and companies in the field of tourism are willing to help to ensure a positive environment for all of their customers and guests.

- When staying in a hotel, it is a good idea to call ahead and ask for a quiet room. You may wish to explain about the person's behavior if there is a likelihood of her exhibiting such behavior in the public part of the hotel. Same with a friend or relative's home; it can be a bit disconcerting for everyone concerned if your child or adolescent takes her clothes off and races through your friend's home stark naked.

- If you are traveling by plane, call the airline as far in advance as you can, and tell them you will be traveling with someone who has special needs. Some airlines have "special assistance coordinators." You may wish to explain about the person's needs and some of the behaviors that may affect other travelers, such as rocking in their seat. If the person is a rocker, asking for bulkhead seats or the last row of seats on the plane will limit the number of fellow travelers that are impacted by the rocking. If you need assistance getting the person and luggage to the gate, or to change planes during the trip, call ahead and reserve wheelchair assistance. Even if the person does not need a wheelchair, this guarantees that someone will be waiting for you and available to assist you. (This was suggested to me by a special assistance coordinator when I told her that the help I had requested had not been provided on a recent trip). When requesting the wheelchair, you may need to explain about the person's autism. For example, I have explained in the past that my son with autism had difficulty moving forward in a purposeful manner and we needed help to get to the gate to catch a connecting flight.

- Persons with autism should always carry identification. Make sure she has an ID tag attached to her somewhere, with a current phone number written on it. You can order medical bracelets, necklaces, and tags to attach to shoelaces. Additionally, if the person can carry it in her pocket, make an ID card with a current photo, date, and phone numbers. Be sure to include any other important information, such as allergies and medications, and any special information (i.e. nonverbal).

- Adult passengers (eighteen and over) are required to show a US federal or state-issued photo ID that contains the following information: name, date of birth, gender, expiration date, and a tamper-resistant feature in order to be allowed to go through the checkpoint and onto their flight. Acceptable identification includes: driver's license or other state photo identity card issued by the Department of Motor Vehicles (or equivalent) that meets real ID benchmarks (at time of writing, all states are currently in compliance).

Chapter 10
Holidays, Birthdays, Gifts

Tips for Surviving the Holiday Season

The winter holidays and celebrations can be difficult for children on the spectrum and their families. Some areas of difficulty include:

- The stores are full of noise, lights, lots of people, and winter holiday music that can create major overwhelm for those with sensory processing challenges.
- Social requirements such as visiting relatives wanting a hug or a kiss that can feel painful.
- Holiday dinners where she is expected to try foods or sit for long periods of time with so many people and so much commotion.
- Many children are mesmerized by the colors and textures of the ribbon and wrapping paper and do not open the present but stim on (get engrossed in playing with) the wrapping.
- The child does not understand personal space or have notions of safety and so she may run around the house or handle something breakable.
- Relatives may think the that the child is misbehaving, and may try to discipline the child, not realizing that

the child really can't help it, and that discipline is not helpful when it comes to sensory overload and high anxiety.

- Parents have a difficult time because they know there are certain expectations of behavior that relatives and friends have and that the child cannot fulfill.

~

What can you do? Here are some tips on how to prepare your friends and relatives whom you will be visiting:

- Explain the difficulties your child has with the holiday dinner environment, decorations, noise etc.
- Let your friends and relatives know that she is not just misbehaving, and that she is learning little by little how to handle these situations.
- Explain about dietary challenges so they don't expect her to eat what everyone else is eating.
- Ask if there is a quiet room (child-proof in terms of décor) where your child can retreat for some quiet time to escape the commotion and noise.
- Send them a short but sweet letter or email explaining why your child acts the way she does and the difficulties of the holidays from her point of view. They will have a better understanding of why she won't wear a dress, and why, as more and more people start arriving, she tries to escape the room.

CHAPTER 11

The Future: Happy 18th Birthday— Where Do We Go from Here?

When you daughter turns eighteen, she is a legal adult, regardless of her autism. You'll need to think about what steps to take to help her make safe decisions about her finances, health, and general living. For some families, but certainly not all, guardianship is necessary. Even though you are Mom and Dad, you still have to become legal guardian for your child in order to sign paperwork and make legal decision for her. If your daughter has Asperger's, you might need Power of Attorney to assist her, while maintaining her autonomy. Consult with an attorney and visit the Autism Speaks Family Services pages for more info. Here are a few definitions:

- **Guardianship** is a court-ordered arrangement in which one person is given the legal authority to make decisions on behalf of another person whom a court has deemed to be "incapacitated." The guardian's decision-making authority extends to all areas specified by the court.
- **Limited Guardian:** A limited guardian makes decisions in only some specific areas, such as medical care. Limited guardianship may be appropriate if the

person with a disability can make some decisions on his or her own.

- **General Guardian:** A general guardian has broad control and decision-making authority over the individual. General guardianship may be appropriate if the person has a significant intellectual disability or mental illness and, as a result, is unable to meaningfully participate in important decisions that affect him or her.

- **Conservator:** A conservator manages the finances (income and assets) of a person with a disability. A conservator has no authority to make personal decisions (medical, educational, etc.) for the person whose funds he or she is managing.

From http://www.autismspeaks.org/family-services/tool-kits/transition-tool-kit/legal-matters.

Transition Planning

The following tips for parents whose children have been served through IEPs or 504 plans are adapted from Michelle Garcia Winner, "Parenting through to Adulthood," socialthinking.com.

Don't wait until the legal age of the school's transition plan to start transitioning your child into increasing responsibility and independence. The kids will not willingly go along with this plan to do more, but set an expectation and reward small (very small) steps toward the accomplishment. Don't overly focus on the sneer on their face or the less-than-complimentary words they may say; pick your battles carefully. Subtly praise any step toward being a more responsible member of the family. Withhold treats (video games, cell phones, books, etc.) if they are not trying to be a reasonable member of the house most of the time. To give in to their stormy ways is to reinforce the cloud hanging over your house.

~

The adult world is unaccommodating—a fact that is hard to face for everyone, but particularly when our special education teams have tried to serve our kids by accommodating to their disability (to some extent). Prevent the IEP team and yourself from making decisions that always keep your child comfortable and in control of what he wants to do. As parents of young kids, we work to keep our kids comfortable; now we have to work, literally work, to make sure our kids are learning to be comfortable with the fact that the world frequently does not offer "comfortable" options.

~

Problem-solving is about finding the least painful option, not the one that causes no pain. Problem-solving often does not actually solve the problem! Assure your child, "Yes, you hate the teacher, but you've got to learn to deal with it! You may hate a boss one day!" Parents then need to make sure they don't step in to intervene, to try and solve their children's problems for them. There is a tendency when we identify a child with a disability to make the child's disability everyone else's problem, but by the time they graduate from school, it is totally their challenge to deal with, mostly on their own. While there will be some special people to reach out and continue to help, especially while they are in their young twenties, the "game" has changed significantly. Our kids are expected to do much more for themselves the year after they graduate from high school than the year before. Plan for this ahead of time!

~

Avoid burnout. Something the parents of my clients have taught me over the years is that they wear out! Begin to work on all of the above slowly but surely when your child is thirteen, fourteen, fifteen. They may have been happy to drive their child to high school, but they no longer want to drive their child to college or their job, nor should they! The social rules have changed, and it is so incredibly unhip to be driven around by your parents when you are a young adult. You won't regret it. Your child won't be ready to fly solo (very likely) by the time they graduate from high school (nor were my daughters!), but they will be more on their way and slowly be able to handle the growing pressures of having to do more for themselves, even if they don't want to.

Some people on the more able end of the spectrum learn to drive. however, it may take longer to learn because of their sensory processing and motor coordination challenges. The easy part tends to be learning the rules involved in driving.

Getting a Job

The following tips are from Denise Zangoglia, "8 Top Tips-Planning for Life after High School for Your Autistic Child," EpilepsyMoms.com, www. epilepsymoms.com/disease/autism/8-top-tips-planning- life-after-high-school-your-autistic-child. html.

Make sure your child takes a career assessment test for some initial direction that can help the student focus on the concrete rather than the abstract. It's imperative to stay involved and keep on top of the process even if you think the school is handling it. Look into options on your own. Some agencies, such as the Department of Vocational Rehabilitation, Social Security Administration, or independent and supported living centers, might provide training or direct services to assist the school with a student's transition. Local public schools are required by law to supply information about these services as part of transition planning in high school.

~

There should be a master plan with short- and long-range goals and the tasks or activities that are required to achieve those goals. The goals and services will be dependent on the needs, skills, and personal preferences of each child. Parents can help their son or daughter by assigning some chores or arranging for volunteer work to discover whether or not they want a structured work environment or a competitive job. The options to consider for post-high school life are:

- Vocational training
- Community interaction and participation
- Level of independent living skills
- Adult services offered
- Postsecondary education
- Adult and continuing education
- Integrated and/or supported employment

~

Consider your child's strengths and interests and don't discount splinter skills (strengths that might be out of proportion to their other skills). Focus on those, as they can be the foundation for thriving in continuing education, employment, and socialization. This can range from careers as musicians, mathematicians, artists, structural designers with mechanical or spatial skills; mathematical calculation skills, athletic performance; and computer ability.

~

Ask career/vocational questions. It's important that the parents, the child, the teachers, siblings, and other significant persons in your child's life be a part of this, as each can offer valuable insights. Some questions to start the ball rolling are listed below, and in the course of asking them, other questions that are pertinent will come up. Add to and refine your list as you go through the process to develop the best direction for your child.

- What does your son/daughter like to do?
- What can they do?
- What needs to be explored more?
- What skills or information does your son/daughter need to learn and understand to reach their goals?
- How does college fit in the picture for them? Four-year, community, vocational, or adult education?
- What options/services are available for learning about employment and/or training?
- Where will your son/daughter live?

- How does a job sound to your child, either supportive or competitive?
- How will they support themselves?
- How will they acquire health insurance?
- Will your child require help and support from you? (You might want to see an attorney who deals specifically with special needs trusts, if this is the case)
- What kind of transportation is available for your child?

~

Ask social interactive questions. Life after high school must also take into account the social network of your child. Friends, community, and a sense of belonging are just as important factors.

- Does your child have the skills to form and foster friendships, or will they need help and encouragement?
- Is your child known in the community through volunteer, sports, creative arts, or religious affiliations?
- Does your son or daughter have a hobby or passion? Are they involved in a horseback-riding program, music program, or club that others might share an interest in as an activity?
- What venues are available for socializing? For example: choir, sports/team recordkeeping/

statistician, religious affiliations, senior center involvement, fire department volunteer helper.

~

Take action. As with anything, planning is not enough. Follow-through is key to a successful venture. If your child is especially gifted with math or computer skills, see if you can arrange to acquire a position for them in a data services job. They will learn the office and social skills and procedures appropriate for a work environment. This might involve clocking in or following a scheduled work task list, or even giving them the right amount of time to get to work on time. Making sure your child can sit for certain length of time required in a work environment is crucial.

~

Try to offer them the tools to help them decide if this environment is one they might want to explore. You might also consider setting up a section of your home or home office for them as a practice work environment. My sister-in-law did this for her child to acclimate him to a simulated work environment. She furnished it with the necessary technology, as well as furnishings such as a desk, ergonomic mesh chair, and photos of the things he loved to make him feel comfortable.

~

Many businesses offer employment in different capacities, such as packaging companies that require assembly with a requirement for accuracy and a deadline, and uniform service companies that require sorting and cleaning. US military installations are very supportive by offering positions that involve copying, folding, sealing, and mailing newsletters. The skills needed and required are neatness and completion of tasks in a timely manner.

It is important that high-functioning autistics and Asperger's syndrome people pick a college major in an area where they can get jobs. Computer science is a good choice because it is very likely that many of the best programmers have either Asperger's syndrome or some of its traits. Other good majors are: accounting, engineering, library science, and art, with an emphasis on commercial art and drafting. Majors in history, political science, business, English, or pure math should be avoided. However, one could major in library science with a minor in history, but the library science degree makes it easier to get a good job.

—Temple Grandin, PhD, author of
Thinking in Pictures and *The Way I See It*,
www.autism.com/ind_choosing_job.asp

~

A person with Asperger's syndrome or autism has to compensate for poor social skills by making themselves so good in a specialized field that people will be willing to "buy" their skill even though social skills are poor. This is why making a portfolio of your work is so important. You need to learn a few social survival skills, but you will make friends at work by sharing your shared interest with the other people who work in your specialty. My social life is almost all work-related. I am friends with people I do interesting work with.

—Temple Grandin, PhD, author of
Thinking in Pictures and *The Way I See It*,
www.autism.com/ind_choosing_job.asp

Attending College

The following tips are provided by Lars Perner, PhD (www.AspergersSyndrome.org).

Choosing a College

- It is tempting to consider getting a start at a community college (CC) rather than at a university, and there are situations where this may be useful.
- Temple Grandin—a hero to many of us!—has very insightfully recommended that high school students with special interests and/or greater advancement in certain subjects take courses at a CC during the school year and/or over the summer. If the student is already familiar with the CC that way, the transition may be smoother. . . . A CC may also be located more conveniently, allowing the student to live at home, or at least closer to home.

- The quality of instruction at both CCs and four-year colleges varies widely, so it is difficult to say whether substantive learning will suffer. Students will probably get more individual attention at a community college than they would at a research-oriented university where many of the freshperson and sophomore courses are taught in the infamous 400-student lecture halls.

- One option is to consider a technical program, or trade school, rather than a traditional university education. Here, the student will have the opportunity to focus more explicitly on his or her interests.

- Many private colleges provide significantly smaller classes and more individual attention. However, the price tag can be quite prohibitive.

- A number of public, teaching-oriented universities may provide a good solution. I was fortunate to go to the Cal Poly, which provided an excellent quality of education. A guidance counselor may be able to offer some good advice on available options within an acceptable distance from home.

Securing Needed Services

- Individuals with autism vary tremendously in the help and services they will need to function effectively, and colleges differ a great deal in what they offer.

- The issue arises as to how much a student should disclose to his or her professors, and what, if any, accommodations he or she should request. This is an individual matter, and the answer will vary depending on the individual case and the student's relative desire for privacy. Theoretically, in the United States, the Americans with Disabilities Act requires educational institutions and employers to provide the disabled with "reasonable accommodations." In practice, however, the act has been described as lacking "teeth" and exactly what it mandates is not at all clear. Many universities explicitly require that any special accommodations must be requested through the disabled student services office rather than directly to a professor. The type of campus involved is likely to make a significant difference. Faculty in small liberal arts colleges are likely to be a lot more accommodating than those in big research institutions, where teaching and individuals are more likely to be seen as obstacles to research.

- Most colleges offer some counseling services, which are often quite in demand among a large proportion of students struggling to adjust to various phases of college life. These counseling services may or may not have staff experienced in dealing with students on the spectrum and even when they do, students may be eligible for only a small number of sessions. University health centers vary somewhat in what kinds of required medial services they may offer.

Moving Away to College and Pragmatics

- For some students on the spectrum, academics are the easy stuff, and the real trouble involves moving away from home and coping with the pragmatics of independent and group living.
- For those going to a college "far away" (a term that will have different meanings to different people), one of the problems is that the transition is so abrupt. You leave one day, arriving perhaps a week before the start of the term. And many of the other pressures are likely to start.
- If a student is within driving distance, feels comfortable driving, and has a car, he or she can have the assurance of being able to come home— if he or she feels the urge to do so—every weekend if need be. The beauty of a safety net is that its existence does not mean thatit actually has to be used—but it can go a long way in quelling anxiety. . . . For those who live farther away from home, open-ended bus, train, or plane tickets or vouchers, for those who can afford them, can provide a real sense of security.
- One very important issue is living arrangements. It is easy to visualize how

disastrous a residence hall can be to an individual with autism. Having to share a room with someone else (a reality in most residence halls), lack of privacy in bathrooms, and the crowded and noisy quarters sound quite hellish, and I am glad I never had to go through that experience. Cafeteria food may or may not be a problem. At least there is frequently a lot of choice, and you don't have to prepare the food yourself.

Special Needs Trusts

We have special needs trusts for the girls, but not because my husband and I are great planners. We aren't. Well, he is, but I'm a classic foot dragger. However, we had criminal and civil cases involving the (non-sexual) assault of our youngest daughter that lead to a small settlement. We had to open a special needs trust because of the settlement. And we got a group rate on three . . . Our attorney was the Probate Judge who had handled Mia's guardianship, and he works just a hop, skip, and a jump from our home. He was expert in setting up the Special Needs Trusts.

~

SNTs serves two primary functions: first, it provides management of funds for your child should she not be able to do so herself, and second, it preserves your daughter's eligibility for public benefits, including Medicaid, SSI, or any other program. You create a SNT to ensure the financial wellbeing of your daughter in the future when you are no longer around.

- The SNT allows you to leave resources for her benefit without cutting off public assistance (Medicaid and such).

- It ensures that your other children will not be overburdened with her care.

- The SNT will make sure that any funds left to your daughter will be properly managed and distributed.

- It provides fair allocation between your kids.

- You may think you do not need a SNT currently, but remember that things change; public programs change over the years, and siblings may have their own difficulties. A SNT can provide a secure future for your daughter.

- To create the SNT you will need the help of a lawyer with experience in SNTs. Ask other parents for references; contact your Medicaid coordinator, as these organizations sometimes provide discounted or free legal help. Ask your current lawyers covering other areas of your life for a referral.

- Your legal help should be able to recommend a financial planner, or you can select your own.

- Together with your legal and financial advisors, you will choose an appropriate trustee who will manage the SNT.

- When meeting with the above professionals, assess your current situation, analyze the impact of the plan on your estate and aid programs, and then adjust as necessary.

Chapter 12

Finances

Autism is ridiculously expensive, as you well know. So many therapies remain inadequately covered, or not at all covered by insurance, even as pediatric preexisting conditions have been eliminated by the Affordable Care Act. Even revamping your household diet to an organic, possibly gluten-free menu puts a strain on the family budget.

My husband went through a protracted period of job insecurity. We were dead, dirt broke for many years, we bounced back before a major account loss plunged us further back into the poorhouse than we thought possible. Money worries are horrifically stressful, embarrassing, and isolating.

In Connecticut, we have a fairly well funded Department of Disability Services. After three years on a wait list, my girls were accepted into a program and received budgets through the state. Our program is not based on income, rather on the LON "Level of Need" of the child. I am able to self-hire staff for both respite and In-Home Services. Acceptance into this program put the girls onto the Medicaid Waiver. My girls need help. I cannot fund their programming myself. DDS has been a Godsend for us. Our program has a legal liability—if we were to earn a whole lot of money, we might have to pay back some of the budget. I'm not worried at this point! Even so, the access to a top-notch behaviorist and case manager who is helping us prepare for adult programming would be worth every penny.

I scratch my head that many families refuse to take advantage of the services for which their kids might qualify. It's not a handout. Your daughter may qualify for programs that will free up money for you and give you time for yourself. Contact your state's DDS office to see if you can receive support.

SILVER DOLLAR PANCAKES

Pancakes are a budget-friendly meal for breakfast, lunch, or dinner, are a pinch-hit for bread, and are great for dipping into hummus at snack time. There are several gluten-free boxed mixes that are easier to make than scratch. King Arthur Flour pancake mix makes a classic, thin and springy diner pancake. Even old Betty Crocker GF Bisquik turns out a spectacular, fluffy pancake, though the ingredients aren't quite as good as King Arthur in my opinion.

Tax Season—Christmas in April?

Tax Tips by Kim Mack Rosenberg and Mark L. Berger, CPA

Disclaimer: The information contained herein is for informational purposes only and does not substitute for tax advice from your own tax adviser, familiar with your financial information. While they have endeavored to be as accurate as possible, the authors make no warranties, express or implied, concerning the information contained herein. As always, official sources and publications and your own tax professional should be consulted for the most current rules and regulations that may be applicable to you.

Medical expenses above the first 7.5 percent of your adjusted gross income are tax-deductible. Medical expenses up to the first 7.5 percent of adjusted gross income are never deductible (even when your expenses exceed 7.5 percent of your adjusted gross income; only the excess is deductible).

~

Save medical receipts for your entire family, even if you don't think you will qualify for a medical expense deduction. You never know when a catastrophic medical bill or a change in family finances could happen and put you over the 7.5 percent threshold.

~

IRS publication 502, available at www.irs.gov, is a great resource to determine what is deductible. Pub. 502 also lists expenses that generally are not deductible, but exceptions in those categories often allow deductions for some of the medical care required by special-needs children.

~

Get a letter from a doctor(s) substantiating your child's need for his treatments and related expenses, like occupational therapy, physical therapy, speech therapy, supplements, special toys/equipment, homeopathy, hyperbaric treatment, the need for you to attend conferences/buy books related to your child's condition or treatment, typical classes (for socialization, for example, if essential to your child's treatment). If you make this an easy step for your practitioners, they are usually amenable to helping you—they want your child to get the treatments he or she needs, too! Keep this letter in case of audit.

~

Supplements that are recommended by a medical practitioner to treat a medical condition diagnosed by a doctor may be deductible, but supplements taken for general "good health" reasons are not deductible.

~

Tuition for a therapeutic school generally will qualify as a medical expense, but if you are reimbursed for that tuition in a later tax year, you will have to account for the reimbursement, and, under some circumstances, some portion could count as income. Reimbursements (including insurance reimbursements) are taxable to the extent that the expense was deducted. If you don't deduct the tuition and then don't get reimbursed, you have three years from the date that you filed that year's return to go back and amend your return.

~

For car travel for medical purposes, you can deduct the larger of the statutory mileage rate (it changes each year and is different for medical vs. business) or your actual expenses (gas and oil, primarily). Tolls and parking are deductible in addition to either actual costs or the statutory per mile deduction. If you use your car in connection with medical expenses and take the standard medical mileage rate deduction, you should keep a mileage log (you can even keep it in the car to be sure to have it when you need it).

~

Conferences fees and transportation expenses for conferences you attend to learn about your child's medical condition/treatment are includable medical expenses; however, meals and lodging at the conference are not.

~

The cost of travel (including an accompanying parent's costs) to another city for medical care is deductible if the primary purpose of your trip is to treat a medical condition. Lodging (at a statutorily defined rate) also is deductible when traveling out of town for medical treatment.

~

However, meals are not deductible (except for the patient in a hospital or similar facility).

~

The *difference* between the costs of foods for special diets (such as the gluten-free/casein-free diet) versus "normal" equivalents is deductible when the special diet is prescribed by a doctor to alleviate a medical condition. For a handy template on these sometimes-complicated calculations, check out www. TACANOW.org.

~

You should evaluate employer-provided plans such as a "flex spending plan," because it gives you the opportunity to pay for medical expenses with pre-tax earnings.

~

Medical expenses reimbursed by a flex spending plan do not qualify as medical expenses for tax deduction purposes—you paid for this with pre-tax dollars and cannot "double dip." (In other words, if you were reimbursed by flex spending, you cannot claim the expense on your taxes).

~

Insurance premiums paid with pre-tax dollars (which is the case for many employees) are not deductible. If you are self-employed, these premiums may be subject to different tax treatment (not as a medical expense).

~

In balancing flex-spending dollars vs. insurance coverage, if you think an expense may be covered by your insurance, submit it to your insurer first. Use your flex spending dollars wisely.

~

Expenses not covered by insurance and not tax deductible may still be eligible for flex spending. These items even include some OTC medications. Consult your flex spending account information on reimbursable items. If you can use pre-tax dollars to be repaid for items that are not tax-deductible, it might make sense to use flex-spending dollars for those items before potentially tax-deductible items.

~

Payments for medical expenses necessary to meet your insurance policy deductible as well as co-pays after you meet your deductible are tax-deductible.

~

The best practice is to keep receipts and to document everything in case of an audit.

~

Documentation of medical expenses should include the name and address of the person you paid and the amount and date you paid, a description of the service/goods provided, and the date provided.

~

Try not to pay medical expenses with cash—credit cards and checks are easier to substantiate.

~

If your child/family has a lot of medical expenses, stay on top of filing regularly. If your paperwork builds up, items may go missing and the task becomes too daunting. Create a filing system that works for you.

Bonus Tips! (at no extra charge)

Submit each claim to your insurer separately, one claim per envelope. Claims are less likely to be lost if they arrive separately rather than in bulk.

~

Keep a copy of the claim form and provider's bill/ receipt in case the insurer misplaces the claim and you need to resubmit, and to help you keep track of paid and outstanding claims. Note the date you sent it on your copy. When you receive an explanation of benefits from your insurer, you can attach it to these documents.

~

Learn how to read your insurer's "explanation of benefits" to determine what is tax-deductible on a given claim and to be sure you are accounting for all potential deductions. any deduction is based on what remains after the charge is reduced based on any agreement your doctor or other provider may have with the insurer, and after your insurer pays its share. These may include: "not covered amounts"; co-pays; deductibles; and co-insurance (for example, if you have a 70/30 plan—your 30 percent share of the allowed charge is a deductible medical expense).

~

To help you and your tax preparer prepare your return efficiently and accurately, create a document (in a word processing, database, or spreadsheet program with which you are comfortable), or use a money management program that allows you to track the expenses by category or groups of categories. If you create a document, you can use the same document and save it as a new version each year—no need to reinvent the wheel.

Afterword

After reading so much information, you probably feel overwhelmed. How about a recipe for a good cocktail?

One of my prized vintage cookbooks belonged to my Great-Uncle Nick Parrotta, who owned Boston's Gay '90s nightclub in the 1940s. He kept a small, red linen-covered book published in 1945, titled *Cocktail and Wine Digest: Encyclopedia & Guide for Home and Bar,* that had been signed by author and President of the International Barmen Association, Oscar Haimo. Somehow, the book made its way to my collection, and I cherish it.

Here's a simple recipe with a name for what we all want for our girls as they face the challenges of being females on the autism spectrum. Bottoms up!

VICTORY COCKTAIL

Fill champagne glass with chilled champagne
4 dashes brandy on top
Garnish with orange peel

Suggested Reading

7 Kinds of Smart (Plume, 1999) by Thomas Armstrong.

41 Things to Know about Autism (Turner, 2010) by Chantal Sicile-Kira.

1001 Great Ideas for Teaching and Raising Children with Autism Spectrum Disorders (Future Horizons, 2010) by Ellen Notbohm and Veronica Zysk.

Adolescents on the Autism Spectrum: A Parent's Guide to the Cognitive, Social, Physical, and Transition Needs of Teenagers with Autism Spectrum Disorders (Penguin, 2006) by Chantal Sicile-Kira. Foreword by Temple Grandin, PhD. 2006 San Diego Book Award for "Best in Health/Fitness."

All I Can Handle: I'm No Mother Theresa (Skyhorse, 2010) by Kim Stagliano.

Autism: A Holistic Approach (Floris Books, 2002) by Bob Woodward and Dr. Marga Hogenboom.

Autism Life Skills: From Communication and Safety to Self Esteem and More: 10 Essential Abilities Every Child Deserves and Needs to Learn (Penguin, 2008) by Chantal Sicile-Kira. Foreword by Temple Grandin, PhD.

Autism Spectrum Disorders: The Complete Guide to Understanding Autism, Asperger's Syndrome, Pervasive Developmental Disorder, and other ASD's (Penguin, 2005) by Chantal Sicile-Kira. Foreword by Temple Grandin, PhD. Recipient of the 2005 Autism Society of America's Outstanding Literary Work of the Year Award. Nominated for the 2005 Pen/Martha Albrand Award for First Nonfiction.

Autistic Spectrum Disorders: Understanding the Diagnosis and Getting Help (O'Reilly & Associates, 2002) by Mitzi Waltz.

Changing the Course of Autism (Sentient, 2007) by Bryan Jepson, MD with Jane Johnson.

Children and Youth with Asperger's Syndrome (Corwin, 2005) by Brenda Smith-Myles.

Children with Starving Brains (Bramble, 2009) by Jaquelyn Mccandless.

Cutting-Edge Therapies for Autism 2010–2011 (Skyhorse, 2010) by Ken Siri and Tony Lyons

Engaging Autism (Da Capo, 2009) by Stanley Greenspan, MD.

Getting beyond Bullying and Exclusion PreK–5 (Corwin, 2009) by Ronald Mah.

Girls under the Umbrella of Autism Spectrum Disorders (Autism Asperger Press, 2007) by Lori Ernsperger, PhD, and Danielle Wendel.

Healing Our Autistic Children (Palgrave Macmillan, 2010) by Julie A. Buckley, MD.

Healing the New Childhood Epidemics (Ballantine, 2008) by Kenneth Bock, MD.

Helping Children with Autism Learn (Oxford, 2007) by Bryna Siegel.

Other Neurological Differences (Autism Asperger Publishing, 2005) by Lisa Lieberman.

Overcoming ADHD (Da Capo, 2009) by Stanley Greenspan, MD.

Physicians' Desk Reference (PDR Network, 2009) by PDR Staff.

Poor Richards Almanac (Random House, 1988) by Benjamin Franklin.

Son-Rise: The Miracle Continues (HJ Kramer, 1995) by Barry Neil Kaufman and Raun Kaufman.

Stumbling on Happiness (Vintage, 2007) by Daniel Gilbert.

Teaching Students with Autism Spectrum Disorders (Corwin, 2008) by Roger Pierangelo and George A. Giuliani.

The Autism Book (Little, Brown, 2010) by Robert Sears, MD.

The Autism Sourcebook (Harper, 2006) by Karen Siff Exkorn.

Suggested Reading

The Complete IEP Guide: How to Advocate for Your Special Ed Child (NOLO, 2009) by Lawrence Siegel.

The Encyclopedia of Dietary Interventions for the Treatment of Autism and Related Disorders (Sarpsborg Press, 2008) by Karyn Seroussi and Lisa Lewis, PhD.

The Everyday Advocate (NAL, 2010) by Areva Martin, Esq. and Lynn Kern Koegel.

The Hidden Curriculum: Practical Solutions for Understanding Unstated Rules in Social Solutions (Autism Asperger Publishing, 2004) by Brenda Smith-Myles.

The Mindbody Prescription (Warner, 1999) by John Sarno, M.D.

The Way I See It (Future Horizons, 2008) by Temple Grandin, PhD.

The Way They Learn (Tyndale House, 1998) by Cynthia Ulrich Tobias.

Thinking in Pictures (Vintage, 2010) by Temple Grandin, PhD.

Three Times the Love (Avery, 2009) by Lynn and Randy Gaston.

We Band of Mothers (Autism Research Institute, 2007) by Judy Chinitz.

What Your Doctor May Not Tell You about Children's Vaccinations (Grand Central, 2007) by Stephanie Cave, MD.

Index

Index

Index